FREE
TO BE

FREE TO BE

Understanding Kids & Gender Identity

Jack Turban, MD

ATRIA BOOKS

New York • London • Toronto • Sydney • New Delhi

ATRIA
BOOKS

An Imprint of Simon & Schuster, LLC
1230 Avenue of the Americas
New York, NY 10020

First Atria Books hardcover edition June 2024

ATRIA BOOKS and colophon are trademarks of Simon & Schuster, LLC

Simon & Schuster: Celebrating 100 Years of Publishing in 2024

For information about special discounts for bulk purchases, please contact Simon & Schuster Special Sales at 1-866-506-1949 or business@simonandschuster.com.

The Simon & Schuster Speakers Bureau can bring authors to your live event. For more information or to book an event, contact the Simon & Schuster Speakers Bureau at 1-866-248-3049 or visit our website at www.simonspeakers.com.

Interior design by Kris Tobiassen of Matchbook Digital

Manufactured in the United States of America

1 3 5 7 9 10 8 6 4 2

Library of Congress Cataloging-in-Publication Data
Names: Turban, Jack L., author.
Title: Free to be : understanding kids & gender identity / by Jack Turban, MD.
Description: First Atria Books hardcover edition. | New York : Atria Books, 2024. | Includes bibliographical references and index.
Identifiers: LCCN 2023053072 (print) | LCCN 2023053073 (ebook) | ISBN 9781668017043 (hardcover) | ISBN 9781668017050 (trade paperback) | ISBN 9781668017067 (ebook)
Subjects: LCSH: Gender dysphoria in children—United States—Popular works. | Gender dysphoria in adolescents—United States—Popular works. | Gender dysphoria in children—Social aspects—United States—Popular works. | Gender dysphoria in adolescents—Social aspects—United States—Popular works. | Gender identity in children—United States—Popular works. | Gender identity in children—Social aspects—United States—Popular works. | Transgender children—Medical care—United States—Popular works. | Transgender children—Mental health services—United States—Popular works.
Classification: LCC RJ506.G35 T87 2024 (print) | LCC RJ506.G35 (ebook) | DDC 616.85/277—dc23/eng/20240125
LC record available at https://lccn.loc.gov/2023053072
LC ebook record available at https://lccn.loc.gov/2023053073

ISBN 978-1-6680-1704-3
ISBN 978-1-6680-1706-7 (ebook)

Image credits: p. 33 by Dana Simpson; p. 64 courtesy of Daniel Truitt

Contents

Author's Note

Many of the people who graciously spoke with me for this book gave permission to identify them by name. They'll be referred to by first and last name the first time they are introduced. Several people in this book, however, are composite characters. They will be referred to by first name or last name only, and these are not real names. Though their experiences are based on real people with whom I've worked and/or interviewed, the characters are not real people. This allows me to tell you their stories while ensuring they maintain their privacy. As a scientist, I love data. I want people's opinions to be based on science. But I also recognize that cold data can obscure the humanity and emotion that are needed to truly bring science to life. I've spent countless hours providing lectures on the data regarding trans youth mental health, and I often notice that at the end, people don't get it. But once they meet a trans child, things click into place. It is my sincere hope that the science presented here, paired with the stories of these kids—both real and composite—will help you better understand gender, and maybe even yourself, so that we can create a safer and more supportive world. The book may also help you understand some of the intricacies related to gender-affirming medical care. However, please do not use it as a substitute for medical advice. Every patient is unique, and you should rely on your doctors' medical advice over this book, particularly as medicine is ever evolving, and there may be new innovations after this book is published.

Jumping into
the Gender Wars

"If I ever knew someone was gay, I'd shoot them. Gay people don't deserve to live."

I was fourteen when my father said that. The sleeves of his flannel shirt were rolled up to his elbows, and I watched as a scowl burrowed deep into his shaggy brown beard. He was staring at the highway straight ahead, his hazel eyes narrowed and full of a rage I didn't understand. There were two hours left in the drive back to my mom's house. Country music filled the old Volkswagen Golf, punctuated by static from the weak radio reception of rural Pennsylvania.

I sat frozen on the passenger's side. I knew he kept a hand-gun under his seat. And I knew I was gay. I looked down at the oversize khaki cargo shorts I wore to look straight. I turned my head toward the passenger-side window to hide any potential flush on my chubby cheeks. Was the comment directed at me, or did someone driving in front of him seem flamboyant? Did he know I was gay? Was I going to die?

I grew up terrified that if anyone found out I was gay, I would be kicked out of my house, beaten, or killed. I spent years trying to make myself straight. I took a girl in my middle school to an awkward movie date. I deepened my voice and stiffened my gait—two habits that I carry around to this day. I briefly joined the lacrosse team in high school and took a girl to prom. But it never worked. I couldn't conjure up heterosexuality any more than I could conjure up the courage to accept myself. I eventually resigned myself to the idea that I would be closeted, and romantically single, forever.

Frustrated by my lack of progress in making myself straight, I spent countless hours thinking about sex and gender. What did it mean for me to be male and attracted to other men? What was sexual orientation? What was gender? Having suffered the psychological trauma of being told that being gay—something so fundamental about myself—was wrong, I was fascinated by the diversity of human identities and the stigmas attached to them. These interests, along with my hopes to escape Pennsylvania and my childhood, led me to study nonstop through high school. If I couldn't have a romantic life, I'd be sure to have a thriving academic life. With my eyes laser-focused on escaping my situation, I joined every school club, took every early college class I could, and eventually made it to Harvard to study neuroscience. After that, I enrolled in Yale School of Medicine. I hoped that being academically successful would mean I could one day be for-given for the fatal flaw of being gay.

I first came to the topic of how doctors should support transgender youth as a medical student. I had always been inter-ested in writing, and Yale had a famous doctor-writer named Lisa Sanders on faculty. She wrote the Diagnosis column for the *New York Times*, which became the basis for the TV show *House M.D.* I emailed her, and she agreed to meet with me over coffee in the cafeteria.

When she sat down across from me with her coffee, my heart fluttered with intimidation. Her white coat engulfed her thin frame. Her cropped blond hair landed just above the glasses that painted the portrait of a seasoned no-nonsense physician. She got right to it, "What do you want to write?"

I explained that I was interested in how LGBTQ patients do poorly when doctors don't understand them. I laid out a list of potential stories: the gay man whose sexually transmitted infection kills him because he was afraid to tell his doctor about being gay, a lesbian who is too afraid to tell her psychiatrist about the shame her sexuality causes her, and a short story about how doctors support transgender kids.

The last one caught her attention: "I don't know anything about that one." I could tell by the tone of her voice that she wasn't accustomed to not knowing something. "What more can you find out about that one?"

While I started researching how doctors support transgen-der kids, Dr. Sanders taught me to approach the topic as a neutral journalist. Hear every side. Read every study. Unearth every piece of data you can. In between anatomy lab and lec-tures, I spent long hours studying in Yale's Cushing Center—a room in the basement of the medical school library lined with famous neurosurgeon Harvey Cushing's collection of brains in jars. Surrounded by these brains, and the faint pickle-like smell of formaldehyde, I devoured the literature on what doctors thought about the mind and gender, and I found a shocking divide. Poring through dusty books and freshly printed journal articles in the dim lighting of the brain room, I learned that some doctors argued for therapy to push transgender youth to identify as cisgender. They said that gender identity was malleable early in life and that it was possible to "cure" kids of being transgender. They argued that this was good because you could save a person from needing medical interventions and surgery down the line. They didn't say it explicitly, but it seemed clear they were also trying to save these kids from a future of living as a transgender person in a society that treated transgender people horribly. I reflected back: If I could have been made straight and avoided the pain of being gay in a homophobic society, would I have wanted that?

On the other side, doctors argued that trying to force a transgender child to be cisgender was dangerous and didn't work. They thought it would instill shame in the child and lead to anxiety, depression, and maybe even suicide. They noted that the early years of a child's life are important for establishing self-esteem, and that shaming children about themselves during that critical period could do lifelong damage to mental health. Those doctors recommended allowing trans children to transition young, if they wanted to, in a stepwise fashion from the most reversible interventions (changing their name or pronouns) to the least reversible (surgery) later in life.

The two sides seemed diametrically opposed: either support children in their transgender identities, including eventually letting them start puberty blockers and hormone therapy, or try to make them identify with their sex assigned at birth. Each seemed to follow reasonable internal logic, but clearly one had to be wrong. It scared me that one side was causing irreparable harm. But which side was it?

Over the next several years, I met physicians and psychologists from across the ideological spectrum and the globe, listening to what they thought. I also met countless trans people and scholars who shared with me their community knowledge and academic writings.

I jumped on Amtrak each month to visit the first clinic in the United States to offer puberty blockers and hormones for transgender youth. The Gender Multispecialty Service of Harvard's Boston Children's Hospital, nicknamed GeMS, let me spend time with their founder, a pediatric endocrinologist named Norman Spack. A gregarious man with a seemingly permanent smile between his gray goatee, he believed that being transgender wasn't a condition of the brain, but of the body. He explained that for these young people, their bodies had betrayed them. They had an endocrine condition that prevented their bodies from developing in a way that matched who they knew themselves to be. So, he treated with hormonal interventions to correct it. He came to the field after spending time treating unhoused young people living on the streets in Boston, a disproportionate number of whom, he learned, were transgender. He heard their stories of being kicked out of their homes for being transgender. He heard about their struggles with gender dysphoria—a term for the psychological distress that results from your body not matching the gender you know yourself to be. Because no one else in the area was helping them, he convinced his hospital to let him open GeMS. He flew to Amsterdam, where physicians had started developing protocols for supporting transgender youth, and he brought their model to the United States.

In my studies, I also visited Amsterdam to learn from the doctors at the Center of Expertise on Gender Dysphoria at Vrije University Medical Center. While there, I met transgender youth and young adults who were thriving, supported by physicians who supported them with endocrine interventions.

On the other side of the spectrum, I met regularly with Dr. Ken Zucker, the gray-bearded, bespectacled psychologist who led the group that wrote the American Psychiatric Association's criteria for "gender dysphoria," a man who firmly believed that young transgender children could—and should—be made cisgender. He sometimes compared being transgender to a delusion, once asking me, "I had a kid tell me the other day that he thinks he's a fox—we wouldn't make him into a fox, would we?"*

Over the years, I met transgender kids from around the world—some of whom were accepted for their gender identity— and many more who were rejected for it. I also began my own research, using large datasets to investigate what predicts good and bad mental health outcomes for young transgender people. Completing my adult psychiatry training back at Harvard, I cared for transgender adults—those who were thriving because

---

* It's worth noting that by the time I met him, Dr. Zucker supported puberty blockers and gender-affirming hormones for many transgender adolescents. His efforts to push trans youth to identify with their sex assigned at birth seemed to be confined to prepubertal children.

they were accepted, those who were struggling with ongoing harassment and the challenges of getting access to gender-affirming health care, and those who were still navigating the difficult feelings that came from transphobic things they heard from their parents when they were young. After residency, I completed my subspecialty training in child and adolescent psychiatry at Stanford, where I sat with young kids who were exploring their gender identities, and their parents, who didn't know what to do but desperately wanted their kids to live happy, healthy lives.

Today, I write from my office at the University of California, San Francisco, where I direct the Gender Psychiatry Program, our clinical and research program for helping young people and their families navigate the complexities of gender and the way society treats those who don't live up to our traditional gender expectations.

It has been nearly a decade since I started studying kids and their gender identities. The politics of gender have exploded, while most of the research and data about gender identity have remained hidden away from mainstream public knowledge. It's a vital time for people to be educated. The science of gender has huge implications not only for medicine and psychiatry, but also for how we understand ourselves, our children, and society at large. As we dive deeper into the complexities of gender, we often learn a lot about ourselves—that our own gender identities are more nuanced than they appear at first glance. We also learn a lot about society and politics. Now more than ever, gender has exploded in the political arena, with legal implications for everything from medical regulation, to education policy, to sports. Whether you're a parent, a policymaker, a scientist, a health care worker, a therapist, a teacher, or someone just trying to better understand yourself and the people around you, comprehending gender at a deeper level will open your eyes to how we can all work to create a safer, more compassionate society at every level.

1

In the Crossfire

Meet Meredith, Kyle & Sam

MEREDITH

On a chilly day in 2017, I pulled up to a house in a suburban New England town. I was a few years into my medical training and writing a story for the *New York Times* about transgender children and the controversies related to their health care. One of my medical school professors had heard about the story I was writing and told me I needed to meet her friend Suzanne. Suzanne was the chair of the sociology department at a prestigious university and had a transgender daughter who was close friends with my professor's daughter, having met her at summer camp.

I drove my beat-up gray 2006 Subaru Forester into the family's expansive driveway in an upscale neighborhood next to the college. Fall had just begun, and their towering fairy-tale stone home was covered with ivy and framed by maple trees with a collage of yellow and orange leaves.

I crunched my way through the dried leaves blanketing the driveway and found Suzanne and her daughter, Meredith, in the doorway, having heard the hum of my Subaru. Fourteen-year-old Meredith stood five foot four and had long, curly black hair that came down to her chest. She wore blue tights and an oversize hot-pink T-shirt. Suzanne stood next to her, just a few inches taller, with the same curly black hair. She reminded me of the classic professor archetype—wearing a conservative dress, thin-framed glasses, and a gold necklace punctuated by small beads. It was hard not to see Suzanne as a grown-up version of Meredith, as they both stood in front of me with perfect posture and a self-assured poise.

Meredith said that she needed to run upstairs for a few minutes to finish her homework and left me to spend some time with her mom. Suzanne took me into the kitchen and made us all tea, placing steaming cups on a floral ceramic platter. The room filled with the scent of jasmine as Suzanne jumped right into telling me about her experience with Meredith. She spoke with the pace of a professor accustomed to lecturing graduate students who hang on to every word and process with lightning speed. As a novice journalist, I struggled to keep up with messy handwritten notes.

"You probably think this is a huge deal for our family, but Meredith really is doing great. It just took some work for us to learn." I quickly realized that Suzanne had tackled supporting Meredith with the same academic intensity that she brought to her university work.

She explained that when Meredith was in preschool, she always liked more feminine things and spending time with other girls. Around age three, she started wanting to grow her hair long, and she absolutely loved the unrestrained feeling of flowing fabric. She'd often run around the house with a dish towel on her head. Even at three, she seemed to have a "cocktail-party effect" for the pronoun *she*.*

Suzanne went on, "I spent most of my life in liberal New England and assumed that these were just early signs that she may grow up to be a gay man. That didn't faze me. I had the background and understanding for that. Up until she was seven, eight, and nine, she was more or less presenting as female, with long hair, and carrying a purse she insisted I buy her. But she was still using her old name and pronouns."

With time, more of Meredith's feminine interests emerged. On Halloween, she would absolutely light up when she got to dress up like a female character she had seen on television. She always played as a female avatar in video games and wanted to dress in fairy costumes at school. Suzanne, though, is quick to note that this could still just have been the behavior of a cisgender boy with feminine interests. I thought back to some research I had recently read, which backed up what Suzanne was saying. Many such kids grow up to at least outwardly identify as cisgender and gay. But that same research also showed that the more "gender variant behavior" a prepubertal child expressed,

---

* Suzanne taught me that *the cocktail-party effect* refers to the brain's focusing auditory attention on a specific stimulus, while filtering out other distractions. For example, Meredith would perk up and notice when someone said *she*, even in a crowded room with lots of conversation.

the more likely the child was to meet criteria for "gender identity disorder" later in life as an adolescent.*

Later in elementary school, things didn't seem to entirely line up with the idea of Meredith's being a cisgender boy with feminine interests. She would come home crying when the boys and girls were separated at school. At first, Suzanne thought Meredith just wanted to be with her friends, most of whom were girls, but she seemed upset beyond that, in ways she didn't really put into words.

"About a year after the first breakdown in elementary school, Meredith let me know that she was feeling something more than just wanting to be around other girls. She told me she *was* a girl. That was new for me. I didn't know anything about it." This insistence on actually being a gender different from one's birth sex is often considered an important distinction in child psychiatry and a potential distinguisher between cisgender children who are gender nonconforming and transgender children.

"I realize this maybe isn't a normal immediate emotional response, but I started downloading every academic paper I could find about transgender children. What scared me was that there was almost nothing, and there weren't many answers to the questions I had. I had a friend who was a developmental psychologist at another university who I would touch base with periodically to help me unpack the data. That friend had

---

* The research here is complex and has some limitations. The "gender identity disorder" diagnosis from the older version of the American Psychiatric Association's *Diagnostic and Statistical Manual of Mental Disorders (DSM)* didn't actually require one to be transgender and may inadvertently have captured many cisgender people who simply had "gender atypical" interests and behaviors. This was changed in the fifth edition of the *DSM*, with the new "gender dysphoria" diagnosis.

intermittently been interested in the topic throughout her career and was incredible at unpacking what was known."

I paused for a second. In psychiatry, we sometimes worry about the defense mechanism of "intellectualizing"—in which people detach themselves from emotionally charged situations by analyzing them on an intellectual plane. I myself am often guilty of it. But it was clear what emotions Suzanne felt—love and concern. She wanted her child to be happy and healthy, and she wanted to do the right thing. She was searching for answers to help her child.

Her friend turned out to be Dr. Kristina Olson, now a professor of psychology at Princeton and one of the foremost experts in the cognitive development of transgender children. Prior to the time she spent with Meredith and Suzanne, Dr. Olson had always been interested in pediatric gender identity, but Meredith's situation drove her deeper into the topic, which ultimately made her one of the most famous psychologists in the country.

When she first met Suzanne's family, Dr. Olson was an early-career assistant professor of psychology studying how young children develop thoughts about the racial and ethnic backgrounds of other children. When she spent time with Meredith and Suzanne, she saw an incredible child and an academic literature that seemed to misrepresent her experience. It set Dr. Olson on a path toward studying kids like Meredith, which later led her to a MacArthur genius award to continue the Trans-Youth Project, which is following transgender kids from all around the country to better understand their mental health and how to best support them.

Dr. Olson helped Suzanne go through the literature that had been published on transgender children. They found that

much of it argued that most prepubertal kids referred to psychology clinics for children with "gender-related concerns,"
vague though the term may be, grew up to be cisgender and
gay. But they also noticed something peculiar about that
research—most of the kids referred to those clinics weren't
like Meredith. Though the children may have had gender
"atypical" interests such as boys loving dolls or wanting to
only play with girls, they didn't assert their gender as female
with the confidence and assuredness that Meredith did. In
fact, in one of the studies, 90 percent of the children, when
asked what their gender was, reported the sex on their original
birth certificate.

Meredith eventually told her mom that she wanted to use a
new name and female pronouns, and for her mom to take her
shopping in the girls' section. Following the recommendations
from the American Academy of Child & Adolescent Psychiatry,
Suzanne took Meredith to see a therapist to talk through the
decision to undergo this "social transition." It's worth noting
that though this was common at the time, many parents in
recent years have opted not to connect with a therapist when
children are prepubertal, particularly if the child has no mental
health concerns and is in a supportive environment. For
Meredith and her parents, though, this was all so new, and
they wanted expertise and guidance.

Finding a therapist with the proper expertise was grueling,
but a few months later, Meredith had her first appointment
with Dr. Carey. Dr. Carey, a cisgender woman about Meredith's
height, dressed androgynously—usually wearing a button-down
shirt and jeans. She was one of the few therapists in the area
who had experience working with transgender adults and

children. Meredith remembers Dr. Carey immediately put her at ease by approaching everything around gender with curiosity and without judgment. Dr. Carey took a nondirective approach, asking open-ended questions and not making any assumptions about how Meredith experienced gender. She asked Meredith to tell her about her relationship with gender and dove into how it related to gender roles, sexual orientation, you name it. They talked about what it would mean to undergo a social transition, taking on a new name and pronouns and dress. They imagined it together: What would Meredith feel like? How would kids at school react? How would her family react? Would it be okay for her to change her name, then change it again in the future if it didn't feel right to her?

Throughout the time Meredith saw Dr. Carey, Dr. Carey also met regularly with Suzanne to ask how things were going from her perspective. Suzanne noticed that Meredith seemed to struggle every time she had to do a "boy thing," such as when the kids at an after-school program were separated by gender for activities or when someone directly called her a boy.

On the other hand, because Meredith had long hair and was wearing more feminine clothing, strangers would sometimes call her a girl. Each time this happened, Meredith beamed and seemed in a brighter mood for the rest of the day. Psychologists will sometimes use the term "gender euphoria" to describe this experience.

Though Dr. Carey and Meredith had discussed that one can be a cisgender boy and have traditionally "feminine" interests— that never resonated with Meredith as who she was. She felt confident that she *was* a girl. After a year of these conversations, Meredith underwent her social transition. She and her family decided that the beginning of middle school would be a good time. She started using the name Meredith, *she/her* pronouns, and wearing more exclusively the feminine and gender-neutral clothing she preferred. Suzanne sent a letter to the school and another to their church explaining what was going on. Suzanne carried a great deal of social capital in both the church and around the middle school, and the transition was relatively seamless.

Suzanne looked me straight in the eyes and said, "Honestly, I was shocked. It was nearly a nonissue." Other kids at school would sometimes ask questions, but when Meredith explained, they always just said "okay" and moved on. While the kids were unfazed, a few adults did seem judgmental toward Suzanne and Meredith. But they never said anything about it. Suzanne didn't voice it to me directly, but I read between the lines and surmised it was because she carried so much respect in the community that the few judgmental adults were afraid to say anything.

I found myself wondering what would have happened to Meredith had her mother not had so much power in their community. Would things still be going well?

After my long talk with Suzanne, she recommended I sit down in the living room and talk to Meredith alone. "I think she'll be more comfortable if the two of you can just chat. I'll be upstairs. If you need anything, just shout."

Meredith and I took our seats on opposite floral couches in the family's formal living room. She brought me some pictures of her from right after her social transition. She had an ear-to-ear grin in each one. She shared with me that after her social transition, though, she was still scared of puberty. She couldn't imagine her body developing in a way that would betray whom she knew herself to be. She first socially transitioned at age eleven, and Dr. Carey let her know that there was a lot of variability in when puberty began for people, but that on average people assigned male at birth started puberty around twelve.

Meredith remembers crying at the thought of being the only girl in her class with her voice deepening. She had read about puberty blockers, medications that temporarily pause puberty, when searching online for information about transgender people. She desperately wanted one. The problem was that, in the mid-2010s, no clinics in the area offered this treatment. Though puberty blockers had been used since around the 1980s in the Netherlands and the late 1990s at the Gender Multispecialty Service at Harvard's Boston Children's Hospital, no clinic near Meredith's home offered the treatment.

Meredith let me know that Suzanne "went all professor" again when Meredith brought up puberty blockers. Suzanne devoured all the literature she could find about them. They sounded ideal for Meredith. The medications prevented the development of the things Meredith was horrified of: Adam's apple growth, voice changes, and the other myriad of masculine physical attributes that would come with a testosterone-driven puberty. Suzanne also learned that puberty blockers are reversible: if for any reason Meredith decided she wanted to go through her endogenous* puberty, the medication could

---

* I'd like to apologize to readers for using this jargony word. The Oxford dictionary definition of *endogenous* is "growing or originating from within an organism." In contrast, *exogenous* refers to something "growing or originating from outside an organism." I avoid the term *biological puberty* since both endogenous puberty and exogenous puberty (induced by taking estrogen pills or testosterone injections, for instance) involve biological processes.

be stopped, and puberty would progress. The main side effect was falling behind on bone density, which doctors would closely monitor. When prescribing puberty blockers, doctors also generally give calcium and vitamin D supplements, while encouraging exercise, all of which can improve bone density. But Meredith and Suzanne still faced a major problem—no doctors in their area had any experience prescribing puberty blockers for transgender adolescents.

Suzanne ultimately reached out to a nearby pediatric endocrinologist named Dr. Stenton and told her about Meredith's situation. A close friend, Dr. Stenton agreed to learn the protocol for using these medications for transgender youth and make it happen for Meredith, in collaboration with Meredith's therapist, who at that point was quite clear that endogenous puberty would be disastrous for Meredith's mental health.

Meredith started puberty just after her twelfth birthday. Endocrinologists use something called Tanner staging to describe the progression of puberty. The first stage of active puberty is called Tanner Stage 2. For adolescents assigned male at birth, this includes growth of the testicles and early development of pubic hair. For those assigned female at birth, it is characterized by the development of breast buds and areolar growth.

As predicted, soon after puberty began, Meredith started to have panic attacks about the way her body was changing, and Dr. Stenton quickly offered the puberty blocker that she and Meredith's family had spoken about extensively over the past year or so. Dr. Stenton coordinated with Meredith's therapist and had the puberty-blocking implant placed before any obvious signs of her endogenous puberty appeared.

Back in her family's living room, about a year and a half after the puberty blocker was placed, Meredith told me more about the medication. Sitting across the couch from me, she rolled up her sleeve and told me to feel around her biceps, where a hard rod sat just beneath her skin and slowly released the medication into her bloodstream to turn off the brain cells that would otherwise kick off the chemical changes in her body that would cause hair growth, voice deepening, and the other changes of her endogenous puberty. The rod felt just like the Nexplanon implant many people I knew used for birth control.

As we'll hear more later, she told me that the blocker was amazing, but she was eager to start estrogen soon. "I'm tired of being the only girl in my grade who looks like a little kid." As she squinted ever so slightly with annoyance, she told me it was awkward that other girls in her class were "developing," and she wasn't. She felt out of place looking prepubertal.

But aside from that, she was happy. She had straight A's. She was starring in her school's production of *Annie*. Two boys had also asked her out that year. She told me she turned to one and said, "You know I'm trans, right?" He looked her in the eyes and answered, "Yes, Meredith, I know you're trans. I also know you're pretty and smart. Will you go to this dance with me?"

Watching her blush as she told me this story, I thought back to the other transgender teenagers I'd met who weren't allowed to transition. So many struggled with low self-esteem, self-hatred, and depression. They were often in and out of the hospital for having suicidal thoughts. But Meredith was thriving. It was beautiful to see this was possible. But clearly much of this was because she had Suzanne's resourcefulness, socioeconomic privileges, academic access, and unique ability to gather experts and medical professionals to make it all happen.

After finishing my tea and chatting with Meredith a bit more, I thanked her and Suzanne for taking the time to talk to me and got back in my Subaru.

Driving home, I felt a strange mix of emotions. Part of me felt light and hopeful—Meredith was doing so well, and her affirming environment had let her thrive. But I also felt a pang in my stomach I didn't quite understand. I found myself digging my nails into the steering wheel and rolling down the window to cool myself down. Just beneath the happiness I felt for Meredith was sadness and anger around my own childhood. I thought about how I never had that unconditional love and support and how much that hurt. I still carry that pain around every day. It impacts my self-esteem and my ability to love myself. I started thinking about the other trans kids around the country, most of whom didn't have the kind of support Suzanne was able to give Meredith. All kids deserved the kind of love, dedication, and support that Meredith was receiving. Whether it's about gender or something else entirely, being listened to and respected has a huge positive impact on a child. The relationships we have with our parents often dictate our adult self-esteem and what our future relationships look like. If we are loved and respected by our parents, we feel more comfortable in relationships in the future and can provide that same love and respect to others. In contrast, if we grow up feeling shamed and misunderstood, we often become anxious in future relationships, which leads to conflict and insecurity. Though negative experiences with parents can be mitigated by later therapy and positive relationships, supportive family experiences are among the most robust predictors of good adult mental health.

Meredith's story was a beacon of hope, but we were still so far away from it being the norm. A few years later, while on call as a child and adolescent psychiatry fellow at Stanford, I would be woken up for a story that sadly was much more typical.

KYLE

At three in the morning, I heard my cell phone blare with the chime of my pager. It was my night on call to cover psychiatric emergencies at the hospital. To this day, every time I get a page, my heart sinks and starts to pound. I get nauseated. My body has visceral memories of every awful thing I've heard with each page.

I called the pediatrics resident who wanted to talk to me, and she told me that a sixteen-year-old had been brought to the emergency room by his parents after an attempt to end his life. She needed me to evaluate if he met criteria for an involuntary psychiatric hold (a legal order placed by a physician that holds a patient in the hospital for up to seventy-two hours during a mental health emergency). These holds are usually placed in the emergency room to keep a patient there until the person can be transferred to a secure inpatient psychiatric unit for ongoing care, supervision, and support. Before hanging up, she added, "He's trans."

I met Kyle and his parents in a small bay in the emergency room. A security guard sat outside the room, standard protocol for when doctors are worried people may hurt themselves or someone else.

Kyle was resting on a hospital gurney with an IV connected to his arm. He was shorter than most boys his age, and his bangs were gelled straight up toward the sky. He wore a black concert hoodie that covered his thin frame, which I eventually learned was because his weight had been impacted by his on-again, off-again eating disorder.

I took Kyle's parents to a small private room off to the side of the emergency room, and they told me more of his story. I learned that in 2008, when Kyle was three, his parents Rosa and Juan immigrated to the United States from South America. About four years after the family arrived in California, Kyle told his parents that he was a boy.

When Kyle told them this, Rosa and Juan were caught off guard; they had never heard anything like it before. They also felt too ashamed to ask anyone for advice. Staying up late one night, they came up with a plan to help him realize what they felt was true: that he was a girl. Over the next few years, they stopped his playdates with boys and scheduled playdates with girls. They enrolled him in a dance class he hated and put him in dresses. They were met with constant screaming and tears, but they never understood why he felt this way. They figured if they just kept pushing, he would come to see what was obvious to them: that he was a girl. They figured that his coming to see himself as a girl would be the easiest way for him to live his life and be accepted. In their defense, there was hardly any public understanding of transgender youth in 2012, and it was unclear where to look for advice. Even if they had known about the academic psychiatry literature at the time, they would have found divergent views, with some professionals advocating for interventions to push pre-pubertal children to identify as cisgender. Not until years later did our research team publish the first study showing that attempts to force prepubertal children to be cisgender were associated with dangerous mental health outcomes, including suicidality.

At around age ten, it seemed as if Kyle's parents had succeeded in their goal. He stopped talking about his gender. But he also became sad and withdrawn. His parents didn't know it at the time, but Kyle had decided to just pretend to be cisgender. The conflict with his parents had become too much to handle.

Over time, his depression worsened. Puberty kicked in, and he hated the way his body was developing. He started exercising constantly and not eating, hoping that his chest would flatten and his periods would stop. As he lost weight, he felt that he looked more masculine, and this made him feel a little better about his body. But the more weight he lost, the more depressed he became. He developed the usual consequences of anorexia—he had no energy, he was constantly sad and anxious, and his thinking became less clear. When he tried to do his homework, he found himself reading the same page over and over, unable to retain the material. Sadly, eating disorder symptoms such as these are much more common among transgender people than the general population. One Canadian study of 923 transgender youth found that 54 percent reported at least one disordered eating behavior.

At fourteen, Kyle fainted in gym class. His parents brought him to the pediatrician, who noticed his heart rate was low and his blood pressure was dropping dramatically when he stood up—signs that his heart was suffering from malnutrition. He was admitted to the hospital, where they gave him more food until he was medically stable. No one in the hospital ever asked about gender, so he never shared his experience with anyone. He assumed he was the only one who felt the way he felt.

After leaving the hospital, he started a specialized talk therapy for anorexia called family-based treatment. In the early stages of treatment, his parents took over control of what he ate and watched him finish his meals. As he gained weight, his periods returned. His body fat came back, and his hips began to grow. He was overwhelmed and panicked by the return of his body's feminine shape, but he was afraid to tell anyone what was going on. While his therapist talked about how many patients with anorexia wanted to look like the unattainable female bodies they saw in the media, Kyle stayed quiet. He didn't want to look anything like that. He thought to himself that no one would ever understand. He felt uniquely broken and alone. Sadly, this is a common experience for transgender youth struggling with eating disorders. Only recently have eating disorder therapists begun adapting traditional treatment paradigms to better support transgender youth and their unique needs, while avoiding the cisgender-focused messaging that's often involved.

Kyle continued to struggle with his eating disorder for the next two years, constantly on the precipice of needing to go back into the hospital due to malnutrition and medical complications. The night of his emergency room visit with me, he was feeling hopeless and impulsively tried to take his life. He immediately regretted it and told his parents, who brought him to the emergency room, where he was now receiving an infusion that would neutralize the toxic by-products of the medication he had taken, in the hopes that it would not destroy his liver. I had sadly seen patients in similar situations who ultimately required a liver transplant.

Luckily, Kyle's liver enzymes (a lab marker of liver damage) eventually came back down, and the pediatricians working in the emergency room said he was safe to be transferred to the psychiatric hospital under the involuntary hold I had placed to keep him safe.* I encouraged the family to have the psychiatrist at the inpatient unit connect with me, so that I could coordinate seeing Kyle again once he was safe to go back to outpatient treatment. Kyle's case was a sad reminder that most families don't have access to providers who are knowledgeable about how to care for and support gender diverse youth who are struggling. And most families don't have access to evidence-based information about how to help their kids. Luckily, with more conversations about trans youth making their way into public awareness, this seems to be changing—something I was fortunate to see with another of my young patients, Sam.

SAM

Sam was raised in Oakland, California, by his single mom, Kate. His dad passed away soon after Kate became pregnant, and it was always just the two of them. Kate was a spectacular mom who was finely attuned to her child. She was closely cued in to what he was thinking and feeling and always dedicated to making sure he felt supported and loved. At a young age, she noticed Sam didn't fit into the gender boxes people expected based on his male sex. In his elementary school, he gravitated to the princess costumes in the dress-up box, similar to

---

* In California, psychiatrists can place what's called a 5150 hold, which legally requires people to stay in psychiatric inpatient care, even if they wish to leave, if the psychiatrist deems they are at an acute risk of harm to themselves. This is a careful balance of safety and individual rights in mental health law. For Kyle, we needed to balance his autonomy against the real potential risk of his passing away from suicide.

Meredith. He asked his mom for nail polish, and she obliged. His chubby cheeks beamed with a wide grin once she helped him finish painting them baby blue. When she asked him about going to have his hair cut, he said he wanted to have long braids down to his shoulders.

Living in Oakland in 2021, none of this caused much of a problem. Kate checked in with the school regularly to make sure it was safe for Sam, both as an African American student and as one who didn't fit into traditional gender boxes. His school was liberal and open, and their philosophy was that children didn't need to be placed into gender boxes. Though most of the kids in the preschool did tend to adhere to traditional gender norms, the few kids like Sam could express their gender however they wanted.

Kate agreed with this philosophy, but when she saw a news segment about transgender kids and medical interventions, she found herself worrying. Was she doing everything she needed to for her child? Did she need to learn more about these medical interventions? Did Sam need a puberty blocker? She loved Sam and wanted to make sure she was doing everything she could to support him.

After doing some research, she found our gender clinic and made an appointment. In the clinic, the first appointment is always with the pediatric endocrinologist. Medications are never prescribed at the first visit, but the endocrinologist describes the range of options to make sure families are informed. The endocrinologist listened to Sam and Kate talk about Sam's childhood, then asked seven-year-old Sam what his gender was. He said he didn't know: "Maybe a boy, maybe a girl, I haven't decided." When asked about pronouns, he said, "I don't care;

use whichever you want." Asked about his body, he said he was pretty happy with it. He especially loved his hair.

During these appointments, the endocrinologist conducts a physical exam to see how far a patient has progressed through puberty. Under current medical guidelines, a child needs to have entered the early stages of puberty before a puberty blocker can even be considered. Sam was still in what doctors call Tanner Stage 1—meaning that no puberty had begun. The endocrinologist told Sam and Kate that there was nothing to be considered medically at this point, but that they were welcome to start seeing the clinic psychiatrist (me) if they wanted ongoing support around thinking about gender, making sure the school environment was safe, and caring for Sam's mental health broadly. Kate accepted the referral.

Because our first meeting was during the COVID-19 pandemic, I met Sam and Kate on Zoom. Knowing that Zoom appointments with young children are a struggle, I braced myself when I logged in and crossed my fingers that Sam wouldn't go running around the house refusing to talk to me.

Kate logged on first and told me most of what she had already told the endocrinologist. I asked her how things were going for Sam in school and in their community, and she said mostly well. The school was accepting of his gender diversity, as were most people in their neighborhood. A few kids had bullied Sam a handful of times, but, from her perspective, Sam didn't seem too impacted by it, and it didn't seem to be ongoing.

I asked how things were going with bathrooms and changing rooms, and Kate said there hadn't been any problems. Sam seemed fine with using the boys' bathroom, where he also changed clothes if he ever needed to at school. He didn't seem to be struggling with any mental health issues—no problems with anxiety, no depression, no sleep problems, and he was eating fine. Overall, he was doing great, and Kate noted that she just "wanted to make sure [she was] supporting his gender development in a way that's going to make sure he's happy and healthy."

After talking to Kate, I spent some time with Sam one-on-one. He jumped in front of the camera with a big smile, revealing a gap between his two front teeth. He was wearing a bright pink shirt with a green turtle on it and cradling a hamster between his arms. "This is Squeakums! Do you want to see my room!?" Without waiting for an answer, he picked up the laptop and ran to his room, carrying Squeakums in his other arm. I saw two bunk beds behind him and asked if he shared his room. "Nope, just me! I just think the bunk beds are fun, and my mom is really nice and let me get them."

He told me a bit about school and said he had great friends there. He said he mostly liked playing with the girls, but sometimes the boys were okay, too. He let me know that he liked playing with the *Frozen* dresses and *loved* sparkly things.

I asked him how other kids react to his sparkles, and his face got more serious. He let me know that most kids at school were okay, but that when he went to his friend Rachael's house last weekend, her friend Joey pushed him, and he fell to the ground. "I don't like Joey." I asked him why he thought Joey did this, and Sam said he didn't know for sure, but he thought it was because he does girl things. "I've never heard him say anything, but I've heard his dad say mean things about my hair and clothes."

I let Sam know that I thought that was pretty messed up and unfair of Joey to push him. Sam's eyes got big. "I know, right!? What a butthead." I let Sam know that this sounded like some butthead behavior indeed, hoping that Kate wouldn't get mad at me for encouraging the use of the term—it seemed fair given the situation.

I asked Sam how it made him feel that Joey and his dad thought this way. Sam said it made him sad, but that "it's a *them* problem, not a *me* problem." I was caught off guard and smiled. It's not every day that I meet a child with that kind of resilience. I knew Kate's open and validating approach toward him had been protective for his self-esteem and mental health.

I let Sam know that I was a special kind of doctor who talks to kids about feelings and gender, and he said, "Cool," thinly veiling that he didn't care and would rather go back to playing with Squeakums. I asked him if he had thoughts about gender or his pronouns. He said he was just himself. He liked using both *he* and *she* pronouns. He maybe had a slight preference for *she*, but didn't particularly care which pronouns people used.

"I'm not really sure if I'm a boy or a girl. I kind of feel like both. Sometimes I feel more like a boy, sometimes I feel more like a girl. I'm not sure it really matters."

It was reassuring to hear her* talk about this with so much ease. We played a quick game of *Pictionary* on the Zoom screen so she wouldn't think I was a total snoozefest, then I asked her if she'd be open to meeting again in a few months. She said sure, then brought the computer back into the kitchen, where her mom was waiting.

---

* I start using both *he* and *she* pronouns here to be respectful of what Sam told me. Following his mom's lead, I wanted to send the message that there is nothing wrong with his gender diversity and that I would respect any pronouns Sam wanted me to use. More to come on pronouns later.

I spent a few minutes wrapping up with Kate and told her that it seemed as if Sam was doing well. She knew about the situation with Joey and said she had talked to Rachael's parents. They had agreed to no longer have Joey and Sam over at the same time, but stopped short of talking to Joey and his dad about their behavior. "I was pretty annoyed with them, but I felt like it was a good enough solution to keep Sam safe."

I saw Kate looking nervous and asked her if everything was okay.

"Is Sam transgender?"

We talked about how some young children don't have their gender completely figured out, and that's totally okay. I reassured her that she was doing all the right things, including the most important aspect for his mental health: making sure Sam knew that she loved him no matter what and letting him be himself. I let her know that most kids like this aren't so lucky. Most are subjected to constant social sanctions for their gender exploration, such as what Sam had experienced with Joey. Sometimes, their parents are the Joeys, and it can lead to chronic self-esteem problems, damaged relationships with parents, anxiety, and sadness. Sam was on a healthy developmental trajectory—he was confident, happy, and loved himself and his family. He got along great with his peers, was doing well in school, and was a compassionate, friendly kid.

At this stage, some parents ask me if affirming a prepubertal child's gender identity will make them more likely to continue to identify as transgender. The question brings up whether wanting a child to grow up as cisgender is an ethical objective (most mental health experts say no). But the ethical considerations aside, it turns out the question has been studied.

In a sample of eighty-five children, Dr. Olson, the Princeton professor who helped Meredith's family, found that the intensity of a child's transgender identity did not seem to change before and after a social transition, during which children were allowed to express their gender identity as they wished.

"You're an amazing mom," I told Kate.

I let her know that there was not much to be done at this point but that she could set up another appointment with me in a few months to check in. I asked her to keep an eye out for any signs of puberty developing, but that for now we didn't need to think about any medical interventions. We could just let Sam be Sam and be open to seeing how things evolved. Maybe he would want puberty blockers down the line, maybe he wouldn't. Maybe he would come to identify as a boy or a girl; maybe he would identify as neither or both. The most important thing was for Kate to just keep being the loving mom she was.

2

A Child by
Any Other Name

Understanding the
Language of Gender

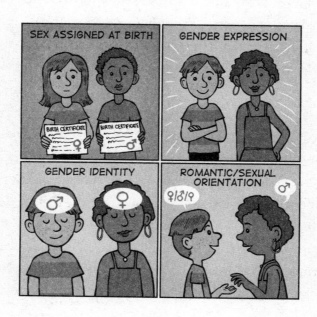

When I meet with families to talk about gender, I often find family members talking right past one another. Kids get angry that their parents don't understand what they're saying. Parents get frustrated that their kids are using words differently from how the parents learned to use them. To make matters worse, families are operating in a political atmosphere that has been making a stressful topic even more stressful. Parents hear politicians talking about "gender ideology" and "mutilating and sterilizing children" and doctors talking about "gonadotropin-releasing hormone agonists." It's easy to get confused, overwhelmed by emotion, and want to run away from the topic altogether.

But I promise that by the end of this book, you'll have the tools and language you need to understand the children in your life, what's going on in politics and medicine, and even yourself on a deeper level. For everyone to get on the same page and find common ground, it's essential we all use the same language, and that we have precise definitions for the terms we use. While the language of gender is constantly evolving, this chapter will give you the essentials to engage with gender in a way that will demystify and create clarity. For families, it's useful to review the terms together, to make sure everyone is using the same words in the same way, so that everyone can understand one another.

Most of us take the language of gender for granted. It's so pervasive in our lives that we barely notice it. But if you stop and think about it, you'll realize you're surrounded by the use of gendered words constantly throughout the day: *he, she, hers, his, man, woman, gentleman, lady.*

Going on autopilot and not reflecting on gendered language is deceptive. It makes something extraordinarily complex seem altogether simple. By diving into the language of gender, we'll reintroduce important nuance. It will help us understand the diversity of people's gender-related experiences and how we can validate and support them. As a starting point, it's helpful to think about three big concepts that people sometimes confuse: sex assigned at birth, gender expression, and gender identity.

SEX ASSIGNED AT BIRTH

Sex assigned at birth (or *sex* for shorthand) refers to what is on your birth certificate: usually male or female. It tends to be based on the genitals the doctor saw when you were born.

Many people think of this as *biological sex*, but that phrase creates a lot of problems. It turns out that there is no single scientific definition of *biological sex*. The term could refer to chromosomes: people think of XY chromosomes as male and XX chromosomes as female.* It could also refer to genitalia: penis as male, vagina as female. It could be defined in terms of internal sex organs: those with a uterus would be female, those without would be male. You might try to define it by hormones: those with higher levels of testosterone in their blood are male, those with more estrogen are female. You may also hear the term *neurological sex*—referring to the sex of a person's brain. For example, a transgender woman's neurological sex would be female.

But these different factors don't always track together. There are thousands of differences in sexual development, in which

---

* Chromosomes are long strands of DNA that live in our cells. Humans have twenty-three pairs of chromosomes in most of their cells. One of these pairs is called the sex chromosome pair. The two types of sex chromosomes are named for their distinctive shapes: X chromosomes and Y chromosomes.

people's bodies combine in different ways. This kind of body diversity is true for hundreds of thousands of people in the United States alone. To give one example, people with a condition called complete androgen insensitivity syndrome may have XY "male chromosomes," but their bodies don't respond to testosterone. As a result, they have a vagina but also testicles inside their abdomen. You can see how the simplistic binary of "biological sex" breaks down. For this reason, scientists who work in the field of gender often use what's on a person's birth certificate and the phrase *sex assigned at birth*—highlighting that this label is assigned to a person based on a somewhat simplistic approach: the appearance of external genitals at birth. But we always keep in mind that it's an imperfect and imprecise categorization.

GENDER EXPRESSION

Gender expression is the way we present to the world in a gendered way. It includes things like clothing, haircuts, pronouns, and names. If I were wearing a dress, you might think of that as a "feminine" gender expression. If I were wearing a tuxedo, you might think of that as a "masculine" gender expression.

These categories vary between cultures, and even across time within a single culture. For example, at the beginning of the twentieth century, the color pink was marketed in the United States as a "boy" color and blue was marketed as a "girl" color. In 1918, the magazine *Earnshaw's* explained, "The generally accepted rule is pink for the boys, and blue for the girls. The reason is that pink, being a more decided and stronger color, is more suitable for the boy, while blue, which is more delicate and dainty, is prettier for the girl." Later in the 1940s, retail companies started marketing pink toward girls instead, and pink became a "girl" color. Around the same time, blue became a "boy" color.

In terms of variability by culture, in the United States, if you wear a piece of cloth that stops at your knees, it would probably be considered a skirt and feminine. In Scotland, a similar piece of cloth may be considered a kilt and decidedly masculine.

We need to keep in mind that someone's gender expression may not always match how you'd imagine they think about themselves and their identity. For instance, some may think that nail polish indicates a feminine gender identity. But plenty of men wear nail polish and still consider themselves men. We need to be careful not to assume people's identity based on what they look like or how we as observers perceive their gender expression. As one physician once told me during my psychiatry residency, "Always be careful not to judge people's insides based on their outsides."

This confusion regarding gender expression and gender identity came up recently for a patient of mine. Carla was seventeen. She was assigned a male sex at birth and was a transgender girl. There was no question in her mind that she was a girl, but she liked to watch baseball and lift weights. She didn't particularly like to wear dresses. When we met for appointments, her long blond hair was usually up in a ponytail, and she wore vintage concert T-shirts and baggy jeans. This threw her parents for a loop. They couldn't imagine how she could truly be a transgender girl when she liked things that, from their perspective, were so masculine. Their confusion was understandable—most representations we see in the media are of transgender people who are stereotypically gender-conforming in their gender expression.

But these media representations don't represent the true full range of human experience.

I asked Carla's parents if they knew any cisgender girls who liked to watch baseball or lift weights, and they realized they had a neighbor just like this. It can be tough if you don't think about it often, but transgender people have the same range of gender expression as cisgender people, and that doesn't make who they are any less valid. Just as we wouldn't assume that a cisgender girl is a boy because she plays with trucks or sometimes likes to wear a suit, we shouldn't assume a transgender girl is a boy because she plays with trucks or sometimes likes to wear a suit.

GENDER IDENTITY

Gender identity refers to one's psychological understanding of oneself in terms of masculinity, femininity, a combination of both, and sometimes neither.

Many people think of just two gender identities: male or female. But we'll see that this is simplistic. Because gender encapsulates so many ways that we think about ourselves, there are nearly infinite ways in which we can conceptualize our gender identities. Gender identity is a complex construct with several dimensions.

On one level, gender identity is something that is deeply felt and can be difficult to put into words. I often refer to this as one's *transcendent* sense of gender. You simply *feel* a certain gender. There's a large body of research showing a strong biological basis for gender identity (more to come later), and this hard-to-put-into-words feeling likely comes from genetic and molecular factors in the brain.

Many kids I meet with describe a feeling of "gender euphoria" when someone uses pronouns that align with their gender identity. It may just *feel right* when someone uses the word *she* to refer to them. Other kids tell me that they draw themselves as a gender different from their sex assigned at birth and are overcome with a feeling that this is who they are.

During the COVID-19 pandemic, many of my appointments moved to telehealth. I spent eight-hour days sitting in my office staring at a computer screen, meeting with patients. One of those patients was Jeremi, a sixteen-year-old trans boy whose parents brought him to me because they were worried he "wasn't really transgender," as they expressed their concern. Jeremi always joined our sessions right on time and sat in a large gaming chair with bright red lines on the headrest that outlined his round face. He had long jet-black hair that came all the way down to his abdomen. Sheets of paper with anime he had drawn served as wallpaper all around his bedroom.

In talking about his gender identity with me, he explained that he thought about himself as a "tomboy" for much of his childhood—a term used to describe a cisgender girl who likes stereotypically male things. He loved LEGOs and wrestling with other kids. Despite this, he had both boys and girls as friends. Many of his girl friends liked playing with the same things he did. But when he went on a summer-camp trip and was told he needed to sleep in the girls' cabin, he felt awful. Even though he knew that girls could like all sorts of stereotypically boy things, something nagged at him that he just wasn't a girl.

One night, sitting on his top bunk in the girls' cabin, he drew a picture of himself as a boy, and an overwhelming feeling of joy came over him.

"This is me," he thought.

To hear him describe it, his entire body felt warm. But within minutes, that joy quickly turned to fear. He could sense tears building up in the corners of his eyes. What were his parents going to think if he told them?

Jeremi's mom and dad are first-generation Chinese American immigrants. Both grew up in Shanghai, where they studied at top universities and became medical research scientists. After years of hard work in pharmaceutical companies there, they eventually secured postdoctoral research positions at universities in the United States. Jeremi's mom shared with me her own experiences of how gender had impacted her throughout her life. Always loving science, she faced a lot of gender-related harassment. In one appointment with me, she recounted how an uncle once told her there are three genders: men, women, and "female doctors," and that no man would ever want to marry a successful female scientist. Having parents who supported her, she was able to ignore this comment, work hard at what she loved, and eventually find Jeremi's father, who was her steadfast supporter. Jeremi's father told me he didn't think about gender much throughout his life. While he was always sensitive to his wife's experiences as a woman in science, he didn't think about his own gender much.

Jeremi's parents were liberal, and his mom's experiences led her to have a broad view of what womanhood entails and a distaste toward gender stereotypes. But the experience of being transgender wasn't something that had ever crossed either of their minds. They grew up in circles where being transgender was never discussed, and most people they knew adhered to traditional gender roles, which were deeply entrenched in the culture in which they were raised. When they first heard about a transgender student at Jeremi's school, they had a strong immediate reaction. After Jeremi's brother told them one of his classmates had come out as transgender, they let out a long speech about how transgender people are just mentally ill and confused. After all, that's all they had ever really heard about transgender people. They had also heard that transgender people had high rates of mental illness and living in poverty, outcomes they would never want for their own children, whom they had worked so hard to raise and set up for successful lives. They told Jeremi's brother to stay away from that classmate. Adhering to their family culture of not arguing with parents, Jeremi's brother didn't say much in response, despite being friends with that classmate. The friend never came to their house anyway, and it didn't seem worth the fight.

After that evening at camp, Jeremi decided to keep things to himself for about a year. But eventually, the pain of hiding how he felt ate away at him too much. He needed to tell his family. He walked into the living room and just ripped the Band-Aid off: "Mom, Dad—I'm a boy," he said, his voice quivering.

His mom and dad, who were sitting on the couch, looked at him with blank stares. He felt his hands start to tremble. They stood up, said nothing, went to their bedroom, and closed the door. For the next few years, they never brought it up again, pretending nothing had happened. As they explained to me later, they were scared and didn't know what to do. They assumed if they ignored what Jeremi had said, things would just go back to how they had been. Jeremi, taking this as an implicit message that his being trans wouldn't be accepted, continued to walk around with a female gender expression, but recounted to me in our sessions that every day felt as if he were wearing a costume. He became more and more depressed and anxious. Eventually, once he turned sixteen, he couldn't take it anymore. He urged his parents to take him to a gender clinic—he needed to talk to someone about this. That's when his parents agreed for him to start seeing me in our telehealth sessions so he could explore his gender identity more; their hope was that by his talking through things, he would come to identify as cisgender.

It's useful to note here that gender therapy is exploratory and nondirective, designed to give young people a framework for understanding themselves. It is important that the therapist not have a "goal" gender identity in mind (transgender, cisgender, or otherwise). Therapy with the goal of making a transgender person cisgender is considered unethical by all major medical organizations, given its link to bad mental health outcomes.* At the time of writing this, it is also illegal in approximately half of U.S. states.†

Sitting in his gaming chair during our telehealth sessions, Jeremi told me that his transcendent feeling of being a male was overwhelming. He felt it "deep in his soul" that he was a boy. When he was treated as a boy, he felt euphoric. When he wasn't, he felt invalidated, unseen, and deeply sad. He described this

---

* Similarly, despite what's said on some news outlets, therapists never have the goal of pushing a child to identify as transgender.

† It's worth noting here that conversion-therapy bans (both for sexual orientation and gender identity) have been challenged in federal courts (primarily using arguments related to free speech rights of those who wish to practice conversion therapy). Different federal appeals courts have taken different stances on this question, and there is reason to believe the question may go to the U.S. Supreme Court soon, potentially before this book is published.

deep sadness as though gravity had intensified tenfold, pulling his entire body toward the ground.

I often think of this deeply felt sense of gender as the foundation upon which we build our gender identities—a biological scaffolding, if you will. But we would be remiss if we ignored the ways in which society drives our conceptualization of our gender identities as well. While biology seems to create the gender foundation, we build upon this foundation with language and experience. This is where societal gender roles and stereotypes come into play. All of us are exposed to them, and it's not reasonable or fair to expect they won't impact us. You may have been raised to think that women are nurturing, passive, and creative. Perhaps you were told that men are assertive, quantitative, and less in touch with their emotions. You probably grew up learning that dolls are for girls and football is for boys. For some of us, these stereotypes don't impact us much. We may even relate to them. But for others, they are incredibly restrictive, maybe even suffocating. Many men are nurturing and creative; many women are quantitative and assertive. Whether we adhere to gender roles or reject them, they color the ways we describe and understand ourselves nonetheless. And their presence emerges even before we leave the womb.

As a fetus, people discuss whether you are a "boy" or a "girl," and these designations may even be celebrated at gender-reveal parties. Parents are set up to have expectations that their children will have gender-related experiences that align with their ultrasound, and understandably, parents imagine a future for their child. As the pink outfits, dollhouses, and fake ovens pile up, parents start to envision what their child's life will be like. Often and understandably, this imagined future takes on a gendered component.

In elementary schools, children are separated by gender, and societal messaging related to gender roles and expectations continues throughout life. Kids see it when they look at adults, when they watch television, and even when they play video games. These gender constructs and stereotypes play a role in how they ascribe language and understanding to their gender identities. While their biologically based gender identity foundation seems to be there from the beginning, these early life experiences are how they decorate and build upon their gender identities and allow them to become more complex. They are also how kids start to ascribe language to their gender-related experiences and how they think about themselves.

The relationship between what kids hear about gender roles and how their understanding of their gender identity evolves likely plays out on both conscious and unconscious levels. The constant messages linking particular traits with particular genders seem to make their way into the depths of our psyches, below our conscious awareness. Psychotherapy often works to bring unconscious thoughts into conscious awareness. This can become important in gender therapy with young people. It universally involves discussing with kids the impact that societal gender stereotypes have on how we think about ourselves, and emphasizing with kids that being cisgender and not adhering to gender roles and expectations is valid and doesn't necessarily mean one is transgender. That being said, because today's generation of young people think about gender with more detail and nuance than older generations, this is almost never news to them.

Many parents ask me if kids are increasingly coming out as transgender because they are unconsciously impacted by what they hear about gender stereotypes. Research, however, shows that with the passage of time, unconscious gender biases are actually softening. In a recently published study, Tessa Charlesworth and Mahzarin Banaji, from the Harvard University Department of Psychology, tested the degree to which people had implicit associations between masculinity and science, masculinity and career focus, femininity and arts, and femininity and family focus. Using data from 1.4 million implicit association measurements,* they found that between 2007 and 2018, these implicit associations have decreased 13 to 19 percent, moving toward neutrality. It's interesting that the number of openly identifying trans people has increased over this period, arguing against the notion that implicit gender associations are driving more people to openly identify as trans. That being said, bringing potential unconscious thoughts about gender into conscious awareness is often helpful for coming to better understand ourselves, and we often explore this in gender therapy when young people express an interest in better understanding themselves and gender.

Parents of my young trans male patients sometimes worry that their children's identities are a result of internalized misogyny. They worry that they "want to be boys" so that they can flee the negative experiences women face in society. I'll often talk to my patients about this idea, not because there is convincing evidence that internalized misogyny creates trans identities, but because it's become a pervasive concept on social media, and many of my patients will be faced with the question at some

---

* Implicit association tasks use reaction time to determine the degree to which people link two variables in their mind on an unconscious or "implicit" level. You can learn more about this technique at implicit.harvard.edu, where you can also test your own implicit associations.

point. I find it helpful for them to discuss it prior to pursuing various types of transition, so that they're not faced with this potentially gaslighting idea during a more sensitive time. But in practice, I have not seen kids identify as trans boys to flee the stigma of being female. They tend to realize that trans people suffer from more negative social pressure than cisgender women.

For some people, rejecting gender stereotypes is even more vital to their gender identity than adhering to them. I often think back to a fifteen-year-old patient of mine named Melissa. I was treating Melissa outside our gender clinic—in a program that supported kids who were struggling with anxiety and depression. Each week, she had a new color streak in her platinum-blond hair: one week baby blue, another week hot pink. She also loved piercings. Her mother worked at a store where she did piercings for a living—it was a sort of family affair. Melissa had several in each ear, one on her nostril, one in her septum, and one on her lip. I would always get squeamish when she talked about the new ones (for a doctor—I'm awful around needles anywhere outside a clinical setting). So, she was sure to tell me each time she had a new one, with an affectionate giggle.

But one day, Melissa said she had something serious to tell me. They told me that they no longer wanted people to use *she/her* pronouns when referring to them, instead wanting me to use the gender-neutral pronouns *they/them*. They explained that they hated the expectations placed on women in society, and they were no longer willing to use pronouns that attributed such meaning to them. They also explained to me that they loved their name and body and had no interest in gender-affirming medical interventions. This was just about gender roles, expectations, and pronouns for them. While some may

feel that Melissa was giving in to misogyny by using new pronouns, Melissa saw it differently—they were empowering themselves and combatting misogyny in their own way.

As a psychiatrist, I'm not in the business of changing
things for people if they're not causing a problem. Though
this may sound minor, it was a major shift in psychiatry with
the *DSM-IV*, published in 1994. In that edition of psychiatry's
manual of mental health diagnoses, nearly every diagnosis was
edited to highlight that a mental health disorder is only a disorder if it is causing problems in social, occupational, or other
important areas of life functioning. It was a move toward psychiatry not inappropriately pathologizing things that weren't
real problems.

While a psychiatrist can give people a framework for deepening their understanding of themselves, the patient is always
going to have a better understanding of themselves than the
outside observer. It's an essential skill, both as a psychiatrist
and a parent, to be able to interrogate ourselves when our kids
see themselves differently from how we see them. Is it because
the young person is lacking insight about something (in which
case, the adult should provide prompts for the child to think
deeper)? Or is something going on with the adult that's making
them unable to see and understand the inner experience of the
young person? As someone who grew up as the only boy in a
house with a mom and two older sisters, I was steeped in strong
feminist ideals from a young age. My oldest sister is a computer
science professor, and my love of science came from her. I was
raised with female heroes in math and science, not male heroes.
I didn't want Melissa to give in to offensive stereotypes placed
on women, and initially it felt to me as if that's what they were

doing. But the more I reflected, the more I realized that Melissa had already considered that. There wasn't something I knew or had thought about that they hadn't. What Melissa was telling me was powerful, assertive, and completely valid. I let them know I would start using *they/them* pronouns and asked them to please let me know if I ever made a mistake. We then went back to our usual cognitive behavioral therapy sessions to help them with their depression. Their depression improved, and we eventually parted ways.

Some families have the urge to refuse to use new pronouns for a young person. Most commonly, it's related to a fear that if they do, their child will continue to identify as transgender and need to experience being stigmatized by our unaccepting society. No parents want that kind of pain for their child. Parents are often concerned that using affirmed pronouns will make this outcome more likely.* Parents may hope that by not using a child's asserted pronouns that the child will identify as cisgender, their trans identity just being a phase. As mental health professionals, we caution against this, as the approach tends to instill shame in the child and damage relationships within the family. Research shows that attempts to force trans children to be cisgender are associated with bad mental health outcomes, including suicide attempts. Beyond that, it also tends to shut down conversations. When teens are invalidated (in other words, told that the way they're thinking or feeling about themselves is wrong), their thinking becomes more concrete and

---

* As mentioned earlier, a 2019 study by Rae and colleagues in the journal *Psychological Science* found that social transition among children does not seem to result in kids identifying more strongly as transgender.

rigid, and they will dig in their heels.* By refusing to use the pronouns children identify as authentic to them, parents who want to open up conversation and better understand what's going on with their child often inadvertently end up shutting down conversation. That can make it impossible for children to be able to discuss and explore their gender identity with nuance.

While relationships to gender roles and expectations may be one aspect of our gender identities, they're not the full picture. Gender identity also involves the way we feel about our bodies. For some people with trans identities, like Melissa,† they are comfortable with their bodies. Many transgender people, however, have a strong feeling that their body doesn't align with who they are. For kids like Kyle, these feelings can be intense and, in some cases, lead to eating disorders, such as the one he experienced. Some feel they should have different genitals or a different chest. Others are intensely bothered by the pitch of their voice or the way their body fat is distributed in a gendered pattern.

Cisgender people often tell me this is difficult for them to understand, yet imagine this: You wake up one morning, and you've started developing all the physical sex characteristics of the other sex. How do you feel? Does it feel uncomfortable

---

* I should note this is also true for adults. Marsha Linehan, founder of dialectical behavior therapy (DBT), has a great module in her therapy manual about validation skills and interpersonal effectiveness. I find it to be one of the highest-yield modules I use in therapy with families.

† Melissa, who identifies as gender nonbinary, also identifies as transgender. While some use the term *transgender* to mean people with a binary gender identity that is "opposite" that of their sex assigned at birth, others such as Melissa use the term more broadly to include anyone who is not cisgender.

when you go to work and other people see you? What about when you're all alone: Does it bother you? How about in the shower? If a doctor told you that hormones or surgical interventions could align your body back to whom you know yourself to be, would you want that?

Dr. Julia Serano, a well-known trans feminist scholar and author of the seminal book *Whipping Girl*, has explained that having strong gendered feelings toward one's body isn't unique to the experience of trans people. In *Whipping Girl*, she describes a thought experiment she sometimes presents to cisgender audiences. She asks them, "If I offered you ten million dollars under the condition that you live as the other sex for the rest of your life, would you take me up on the offer?" In describing the typical audience reaction, she tells readers, "While there is often some wiseass in the audience who will say 'Yes,' the vast majority of people shake their heads to indicate 'No.'"

You may be starting to realize that these different facets of gender identity (relationship to the myriad of gender roles we encounter, relationship to body, and relationship to "transcendent" feelings) can combine in nearly infinite ways. When people say their gender identity is "male" or "female," it's really a shorthand—an attempt to combine how they feel about all these multiple factors—into one label. For people who, on average, feel that these things match up with societal expectations based on their sex assigned at birth, they would probably call themselves cisgender. For people who, on average, feel that these things align with the "opposite" of their sex assigned at birth, they may say they are transgender.

In reality, though, our gender identities are way more complicated. Many people identify as nonbinary, meaning they don't fall neatly into the buckets of "male" or "female." Rather, their gender identities are combinations of both or lie somewhere in between these labels. Some people don't identify with gender at all and consider themselves agender. A 2022 study from the Pew Research Center found that 3 percent of people ages eighteen to twenty-nine in the United States openly identified as nonbinary, highlighting that younger generations are increasingly thinking about their gender in these more nuanced ways.

Most of us are probably more nonbinary than we give ourselves credit for. Because gender identity is so complex and multidimensional, it's rare for people to have every aspect of themselves fall into the "male" or "female" bucket. As you go through this book, I encourage you to reflect on your complex multidimensional sense of your own gender. Feel free to take a moment now to grab a notebook you'll keep close by while reading.

Write down a few words about your gender identity. How do you relate to gender roles? The gendered aspects of your physical body? Is there also a transcendent feeling to your gender identity (if you're struggling with this one, try drawing yourself as male and then again as female—or have someone use different pronouns with you to see how it feels)? If you woke up tomorrow and you had different genitals, would your gender identity be different?

For most people, their general sense of their gender identity doesn't oscillate dramatically. As we'll discuss later, research suggests there are strong biological factors that determine the core foundation of our gender identities. But that doesn't mean the way we think about and ascribe language to them stays exactly the same for people throughout their life. If you're a woman, the way you thought about your femininity when you were in high school is likely very different from how you think about yourself as a woman if you're now a forty-year-old mother of three. Take a minute and write down how your understanding of your gender identity has changed over your lifetime.

How has the way you think about your gender changed over your lifetime? Is it the exact same now as it was when you were younger?

Interrogating our own gender identities can be extraordinarily difficult. On one level, most of us aren't provided with the language and framework to think about this in a nuanced way. On another level, it can be an extremely emotional experience. Most of us are raised to take our gender identity as a given. If you don't experience much distress around your gender identity, you may never think about it. Or you may have been so forced into a gender box as a young person that you were afraid to ever think about it too hard, at the risk of finding something scary. I tend to see several reasons that interrogating gender identity can feel overwhelming.

First is that gender roles and stereotypes have created a lot of problems in the world. Stereotypes about women have been used to disenfranchise them. This includes everything from justifying why women are paid less for the same jobs as men to attempts to restrict their civil liberties like voting. These problems are painful emotionally, and it can be a natural reaction to not want to dive into this painful reality.

Reflecting on your gender identity can also be difficult due to past experiences of *gender threat*. Many people have experiences in childhood in which they exhibit some behavior that isn't expected based on their sex assigned at birth, then something bad happens. Maybe you're a person who was assigned male at birth and played with dolls as a kid. You may have been bullied by kids at school or maybe screamed at by your father for playing with a doll. Maybe you're a person assigned female at birth who wanted to play rugby, and someone told you that no one would want to date a "masculine" girl who plays a "boy sport." Gender threat, especially when it happens in childhood, can make us afraid to reflect on our gender. We may force ourselves to accept societal expectations around gender identity and expression and push down any conflicts we have toward them. Early childhood experiences like these can stick with us, sometimes for our entire adult lives.

We may also be afraid that if we think about it too hard, we'll find something frightening—a gender nonconforming part of ourselves that will put us in danger of that sort of threat again. I see this in kids all the time. Transgender kids will often act in an exaggerated way that aligns with societal expectations based on their sex assigned at birth, hoping no one will ever realize they are transgender. They'll push away every gender nonconforming part of themselves to escape the intimidating possibility of being trans. Sometimes they hope that acting that way will make them cisgender. This can create a lot of confusion for parents, who are then surprised when their kids come out to them as transgender later in life. They'll often think that the transgender identity came out of nowhere when, in reality, it was a carefully guarded secret due to fear of gender threat.

Sometimes, this lasts far past childhood and into adulthood. Particularly for older generations, acknowledging a trans identity can be far too overwhelming to even consider. Part of my job at UCSF, in addition to running our mental health program for transgender youth, is to work as a psychiatrist in our adult LGBTQ psychiatry clinic, where about 80 percent of our patients are transgender. Many of them are people who came out later in life.

One of my patients there, Susan, came out as transgender in her sixties. She grew up in Alabama in a conservative family. She remembers from a young age feeling that she was a girl. She had fantasies of growing up to be a woman, but her father would scream at her anytime she did anything remotely feminine. She remembers her dad even yelling at her about the way she held her books (she held them at her side perched on her hip, which he considered feminine—she needed to hold them directly down at her side). She remembers "butching up," as she described it to me, and forcing herself to present as masculine in every way. She wouldn't even let herself think about being feminine. She went to college, became an IT expert, married her high school girlfriend, and had a child. Eventually, when Susan was fifty and her child was off at college, she and her wife relocated to the Bay Area for a job. Being in a new place where transgender people were living their lives proudly, her deeply repressed gender feelings began to resurface. This time, she couldn't push them back down and was lucky to find a gender therapist in the community to talk through what she was feeling. Following years of therapy, she eventually told her wife, who, to Susan's surprise, was overwhelmed but still supportive. After taking a week to digest the information, her wife told her, "This is big news and a lot to take in, but you're still the person I've loved all these years. I love you like I always have, and we're going to figure this out." Susan eventually started her transition (first with a new name and pronouns, and eventually by starting estrogen therapy) and describes being happier than she's ever been. It hasn't been easy—she continues to deal with the constant stress of being misgendered and living in a society not accepting of trans people—but she describes a freedom that she never felt before. Life isn't easy, but the challenges are worth it—she finally feels like herself.

Have you ever experienced gender threat as a child or as an adult? Write down a few words about your experience and how it impacted you. As you reflect on your own gender identity, do any feelings of anxiety come up? Any anxious thoughts? What do you think the root of these are?

When we see younger generations explore their gender in ways we weren't able to when we were younger, it can also bring up feelings of jealousy or resentment. Many of us were forced to suppress gender nonconforming parts of ourselves at various stages of our lives, and it can feel unfair that younger generations have more freedom than we had. It can be painful to open this back up, but there's extraordinary freedom, authenticity, and liberation to be experienced.

Angelica Ross, who is known for playing the role of Candy Ferocity in the television show *Pose,** recently discussed in the ABC News special *Freedom to Exist* her theory behind why there's been so much backlash toward transgender people in recent years. She emphasized this feeling of resentment that can arise when people see today's generation of transgender people refusing to let society force them into boxes the way past generations were. She highlighted that this isn't just about gender,

---

* While most people know Angelica Ross for her illustrious acting career, she is also a self-taught coder and founded the company TransTech Social Enterprises, which aims to uplift trans people by fostering their skills in the technology industry.

but that there are infinite ways in which society makes us feel constrained, infinite ways in which we are forced, throughout our lives, to act in ways that aren't authentic to how we feel. She explained, "The biggest misconception about trans people is that trans is a choice. It's the biggest misconception because *it is* a choice. And it's hard to understand that when the choice I'm talking about is *choosing yourself.* That's the choice. And you realize that there's so many people who are not trans who are not choosing themselves in their everyday life. That's the jealousy. That's the hatred, is people seeing trans people make a choice to choose themselves, and they can't make the same choice for themselves. I don't mean in the same way. I don't mean that everybody wants to transition, but everybody wants to be free."

I saw some of this frustration come up recently when I met up with a colleague of mine. When he walked into the coffee shop, I could see his wispy hot-pink hair sticking above the person standing in front of him in line. Once he had his drink, he sat down across from me, cradling his take-out coffee cup in both hands. I noticed his face looked serious, the muscles around his eyes tensing. His coffee cup collapsed slightly under the tension in his hands, as if the lid were about to fly off.

"Jack—I'm just so angry."

Over the next hour, he talked to me about how he had been working with his therapist to talk about his gender identity. He'd faced a great deal of gender threat as a child growing up in Indiana. Because he swayed his hips and always wanted to paint his nails, the other kids he grew up with teased him mercilessly. From his perspective, his parents took the bullies' side, telling him that if he didn't change the way he behaved, it was inevitable he'd be teased more. The bullying for his femininity was unbearable. There were times that he was suicidal. He suppressed every feminine part of himself for years and played up only the masculine parts. He became a star football player. Once he felt he presented as sufficiently masculine, he built up the courage to tell his parents he was attracted to men. Initially they reacted with fear and anger, but over a decade or so, his parents softened toward seeing him as a gay man.

But now in therapy, he realized that the gay man label didn't really fit. Having moved to San Francisco, where he could comfortably be himself, he allowed his feminine gender expression to flourish again. He finally painted his nails, something he used to do in secret then quickly remove before leaving the house. He started wearing more clothing from the women's section. And he realized that neither the masculine nor feminine labels fit. He also felt that it wasn't just his gender expression, but that something deep within him felt not entirely male. He told me he was still working with his therapist to understand himself, but he thought he was nonbinary. And he was furious.

"I can't believe I spent so many years suppressing who I was. I went through so much shame. So much sadness. And now I find myself jealous and resentful. Resentful toward society for making me suppress who I am. Jealous of these kids who can live in a free world. One that I didn't get to experience as a child. It hurts so much." He also explained that suppressing himself had deeply impacted his self-esteem. He was constantly unhappy with himself in vague ways that extended beyond gender. Romantic relationships were hard because he never felt deserving of love.

A year later, he shared with me that therapy had helped him feel more comfortable with both the masculine and feminine aspects of his identity, and he had settled into considering himself nonbinary and was using *they/them* pronouns. They'd also begun the journey of reconnecting with their parents. Though they hadn't been able to do it yet, they hoped that in sharing their nonbinary identity with them, they'd be able to be more authentic with them and forge a deeper connection.

NAMES, PRONOUNS, AND MISGENDERING

If you've never experienced someone using the wrong language to describe you, you probably wouldn't think about how painful misgendering can be. Imagine if everyone referred to you as a gender different from your gender identity.

Try this experiment: Tell a member of your family to use the wrong pronouns for you for an entire week. Keep track of the thoughts and emotions that come up each time you are misgendered. Do you feel invalidated? Disrespected? Judged? Does it feel like a comment about your appearance? Your desirability?*

After meeting Kyle in the emergency room, I would later reconnect with him in my outpatient therapy office. During one of our meetings, we talked about an op-ed by a *Wall Street Journal* opinion columnist he had found. In it, the writer argued it was unfair to coerce cisgender people to use the pronouns transgender people identify with. Kyle took a deep sigh and

---

* While going through this exercise, some may experience the gender euphoria that I mentioned some trans children experience when people start using their affirmed pronouns. If this happens, note it as you continue to work through the book and explore your own gender identity.

looked up at me, tears forming in the corners of his large brown eyes.

"She just doesn't get it."

Kyle explained that when someone calls him by his birth name or refers to him with female pronouns, it makes him feel invalidated and unseen. But it also brings up a lot more. It reminds him of the classroom bully who pushed him against a wall when he was walking between classes at school. He remembers his homework sheets and textbooks flying across the hall, and watching as people stepped on his worksheets, leaving dirty brown shoeprints.

Hearing female pronouns also brings up memories of his parents not accepting his gender identity. When someone uses the wrong pronouns to address him, his "Spidey senses" go up. He's immediately on guard. *Is this person a threat? Are they going to physically assault me? Or did they just not know?* It's hard to assume good intentions when his experiences have mostly been bad ones.

Research backs up Kyle's point that language dramatically impacts mental health. In 2018, researchers from the University of Texas at Austin set out to quantify the impact of affirmed names on the mental health of young people. They looked at surveys completed by 129 transgender youth from three big cities as part of the Risk and Protective Factors for Suicide among Sexual Minority Youth study. The study asked these young people the settings in which people were using their chosen name: at school, at home, at work, or with friends. For each additional setting in which a chosen name was used, there was a 56 percent decrease in suicidal behavior. This was true even when they controlled for the impact of accepting social environments broadly.

While we are most accustomed to the gender pronouns *he* and *she*, some people (such as Melissa and my physician colleague) use pronouns to symbolize that they don't feel comfortable in purely male or female expressions of themselves. Nonbinary people often use pronouns other than *he* or *she* because those pronouns feel inauthentic to them. Most commonly, they tend to use the pronouns *they/them/theirs*. You may also hear a range of "neopronouns," such as *ze/zir/zirs*. Just as it may feel hurtful to someone if you use *he/him/his* when that person uses *she/her/hers*, using binary pronouns for nonbinary people can also feel invalidating and hurtful, as though you are trying to push them into gender boxes in which they don't fit.

If you've spent decades taking the language around gender for granted, it can be really difficult to break old habits. Most people go on autopilot with names and pronouns. It can take a lot of effort to slow down and change these habits, but the investment is well worth it to support the mental health of transgender people around you. While it may seem small, it sends a powerful message of acceptance that can be healing for the past experiences of invalidation and harassment many trans people have experienced. It can also allow you to slowly gain trust from someone, bringing you closer so you can better understand the person's experiences.

GENDER DYSPHORIA AND GENDER INCONGRUENCE

As doctors, we have some clinical terms we use when it comes to gender. *Gender dysphoria* refers to psychological distress related to your gender identity and your sex assigned at birth not being in alignment. It's technically a mental health diagnosis, being listed in the American Psychiatric Association's *Diagnostic and Statistical Manual of Mental Disorders (DSM)*, the book that's considered the gold standard for defining diagnoses in psychiatry. Many feel its inclusion in the manual is offensive, implying that being transgender is a mental illness. In reality, being transgender is merely a healthy normal part of human diversity—something the American Psychiatric Association has explicitly acknowledged. There have been extensive conversations about whether the diagnosis should be removed from the manual, much as homosexuality was removed from it in the past. On the one hand, people highlight that the diagnosis is weaponized to imply that being transgender is a mental illness. On the other, people say that the diagnosis is needed for insurance purposes, to ensure medical providers can bill for gender-affirming medical care that many trans people need. I often reflect on the fact that though its inclusion in the manual can be stigmatizing because we stigmatize mental health conditions, the ideal situation would be if we successfully combatted the notion that mental health conditions should be stigmatized. We shouldn't stigmatize major depressive disorder, and we shouldn't stigmatize gender dysphoria. That being said, the sad reality today is that mental health diagnoses *are* stigmatized, and the debates regarding the gender dysphoria diagnosis will continue, without an easy answer.

For some transgender and nonbinary people, gender dysphoria is very closely tied to their physical bodies, and they may be interested in some of the medical interventions we'll talk about later. Other people, like Melissa, who went from using *she/her* to *they/them* pronouns to express their rejection of gender norms, may be transgender or nonbinary but totally okay with their bodies.

Many transgender people have excellent mental health and no "dysphoria" per se. For this reason, it's important to acknowledge that gender dysphoria and being transgender are not the same thing. Highlighting this point, the World Health Organization's International Classification of Diseases (ICD) replaced its mental health diagnosis "gender dysphoria" with the diagnosis "gender incongruence." To meet this diagnosis, one simply must have a gender identity different from one's sex assigned at birth. Unlike the diagnosis of gender dysphoria, no distress is necessary, again highlighting that many trans people who are affirmed and in supportive environments have excellent mental health. The ICD also moved their new diagnosis out of their mental health chapter, working to fight the false notion that being transgender is a mental illness.*

SEXUAL ORIENTATION, DRAG, AND CROSS-DRESSING

There are many terms out there that are often conflated with *gender identity*. The first is *sexual orientation*. *Sexual orientation* refers to the types of people toward whom we are romantically or sexually attracted. We generally use someone's gender identity as the reference point. For example, a transgender woman attracted

---

* In the ICD-11, the diagnosis was moved into the "conditions related to sexual health" section. I'm not sure I agree with this, and I worry that, as Julia Serano pointed out in her latest book, *Sexed Up*, this may reflect society's tendency to inappropriately sexualize LGBTQ people.

to other women would most likely identify as a lesbian.* It's worth highlighting that you can't use someone's gender identity to predict their sexual orientation. Just as a cisgender man can be attracted to men and be gay, so can a transgender man. In fact, research shows that transgender people are much more likely to be nonheterosexual than cisgender people.

Some political pundits have asked whether some young people come to identify as trans in an attempt to flee the stigma related to being gay. They present the theory that straight trans kids are treated better than cisgender gay and lesbian kids. Research doesn't back this up. When we recently looked at data from a national survey of high school students in the United States, we found that transgender kids had much higher rates of bullying victimization than cisgender lesbian, gay, and bisexual kids. Though gender therapists will make sure that young people aren't confusing sexual orientation and gender identity, particularly for younger kids and those with more rigid thinking styles, it's rarely the case that kids identify as trans because they think it will be easier than being gay and cisgender.

Similar to confusion between sexual orientation and gender identity, I often hear confusion regarding the distinction between drag and being transgender. Drag is an art form in which people perform various aspects of gender expression. Most commonly, you'll hear the term *drag queen* (an artist whose performance focuses on expressing femininity), but there are also *drag kings* (artists who focus on expressing masculinity). For

---

* That being said, it's always best to avoid assumptions and ask people the terms with which they most identify.

these people, this is a hobby or their job, not their gender iden-tity. There are drag queens who are cisgender men, drag queens who are transgender women, drag queens who are nonbinary, drag queens who are transgender men—you name it. Drag is about performance art, and it is not a gender identity. To drive this point home, one of the most celebrated drag queens in the United States is Kade Gottlieb—a transgender man from Scottsdale, Arizona. Kade's gender identity is male, and he is a professional makeup artist who performs femininity onstage. He was recently on the popular show *RuPaul's Drag Race*, coming in third place with his signature feminine clown makeup and high-fashion costumes. The next season, the show saw compet-itor Maddy Morphosis, a cisgender straight male competitor,

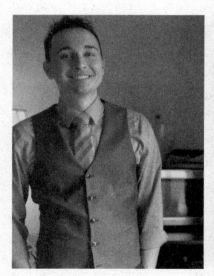 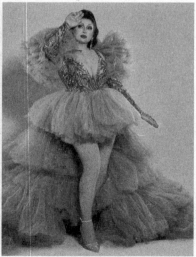

On the left is Daniel Truitt, who is straight and cisgender. On the right is Daniel performing as his drag persona, Maddy Morphosis. Daniel came to fame after competing on the television show *RuPaul's Drag Race*.

highlighting again that drag is not synonymous with a particular gender identity or sexual orientation.

Another term that gets thrown around is *cross-dressing*. This is a broad term that refers to anytime a person wears clothes that aren't expected based on their sex assigned at birth. It's an older term that isn't used much anymore. In the past, it had been used pejoratively to refer to transgender people, in an attempt to invalidate their identities and focus instead on only their gender expression.

You may also come across the term *transsexual*. This is another older term that most people now find pejorative. While some people (including some transgender people who personally identify with the term) still use it to specifically describe transgender people with a desire to pursue gender-affirming medical or surgical interventions, most people choose to avoid it, given its ties to antitrans rhetoric.

Now that we've covered the language of gender, I invite you to reflect on these nuances not just as you continue to read this book, but also in your day-to-day life. Bringing a more refined lexicon and conceptualization to gender empowers us to understand ourselves and people around us, so we can truly see and understand them, instead of shoving complexity under the rug. As we've seen, gender identity is complex and means different things for different people. There is no one way to be transgender, just as there is no one way to be cisgender. The more we open up our conceptualization and use shared language, the more we can come together, understand, and support one another—and in particular our children—in our infinite diversity. This shared language and authenticity can deepen relationships and help people feel seen, understood, and loved. As we interrogate our own gender identities, we can also come to see times in the past that we maybe veered from our authentic selves to flee stigma. Feel free to come back to this chapter throughout your time reading and take more notes on how you understand your own gender in all its complexities. Perhaps you're now in a safer place where you can fight back against that stigma and experience the freedom to be yourself—in your beautiful, multidimensional, complex gendered experiences.

3

Gender Foundation

The Biology of Diverse Gender Identities

Back in 2017, sitting on the floral couches in Suzanne's living room, I asked her what she thought about the nature-versus-nurture question when it came to trans identities. She paused to think for a moment, as the steam of jasmine tea framed her face. "You know, there were signs so early on that it's hard to imagine there wasn't a big nature component." She explained that it seemed clear from a very young age that there was something innate about her daughter that led her to gravitate toward "feminine" things.

Suzanne reminded me that many of the early things she noticed with Meredith she didn't notice with Meredith's brother, who had grown up in essentially the same environment. At age three, Meredith was adamant about growing her hair long, loved the feeling of freely flowing fabric, ran around the house with a dish towel on her head, and gravitated to the gowns in the dress-up box at preschool—especially the fairy outfits.

By the time she was seven, she was carrying a purse, had long hair, and most people she met assumed she was a girl, even though she was still using her masculine name from birth and *he/him* pronouns. All her friends were girls, and she always played as feminine characters in video games. There were plenty of boys in her class she could have associated with, but she never had the interest.

There seemed to be some sort of biological engine driving Meredith's interests and the way she related to the world. When Suzanne tried to take away dolls, Meredith would scream and cry in a way she never did when toy trucks were taken away. Suzanne couldn't think of anything in the environment that could possibly have caused this. And if there were some sort of major environmental "nurture" factor at play—why wouldn't her brother have had similar traits?

Of course, gender identity is more complex than liking dolls, and Meredith's gender identity grew in complexity and nuance as she experienced the world. I'd also be remiss not to highlight that there are many toddlers like Meredith who ultimately grow up to at least outwardly identify as cisgender,* and there are

---

* Research shows that as many as 80 percent of prepubertal children referred to gender clinics at those young ages grow up to at least outwardly identify as cisgender (however, many kids in those studies never asserted a transgender identity, or a gender identity different from their sex assigned at birth—many were likely cisgender kids who had "gender atypical" interests, such as boys who enjoyed dolls or cisgender tomboys). Among children who, like Meredith, did assert that they were a gender different from their sex assigned at birth and pursued an actual social transition, the vast majority, around 98 percent, continued to identify as transgender at least over a five-year follow-up period.

many adult trans people who didn't seem to have these clear hints of gender diversity at very young ages. But certainly, for Meredith and her family, there was something to those innate early gender-related feelings, behaviors, and urges. Talking to Suzanne about toddler Meredith, I found myself wondering, What is it that creates our biologically based gender identity foundation? The answer starts in the mid-twentieth century, with one of the most dramatic stories in medical history.

JOHN MONEY AND THE JOHN-JOAN CASE

Scientists didn't always think that gender identity had a biological basis. In fact, for many decades, including recent ones, it was dogma that gender identity was a purely social construct. The dominant thinker in the field in the mid-twentieth century was a psychologist named John Money.

New Zealand–born Money was a professor of pediatrics and psychology at Johns Hopkins University, where he popularized the idea that gender was purely a result of our social environments. His theories were grounded in his research on children with differences of sexual development—those for whom the various domains of sex (external genitalia, internal sex organs, chromosomes)—didn't all neatly align the way doctors expected. Based on his review of patients in the Hopkins clinic, it seemed to Money that about half of those children were raised as female, half were raised as male, and that they generally seemed to do well. He concluded that it wasn't innate biology that dictated one's gender identity, but rather how one was raised and treated by one's social environment. Writing around the same time that feminist movements were gaining traction in the

United States, his ideas dominated popular culture. Renowned feminist writer Kate Millett even cited Money's work in her seminal *Sexual Politics*, published in 1970. The notion that gender was socially constructed allowed the feminist movement to make huge strides in emphasizing that women should not be treated any differently from men.

One of the foundational pieces of evidence Money used for his assertion that gender identity was not based on innate biology came from his so-called John-Joan case. The story of the pseudonymous child John, who would come to be raised as Joan, began in Winnipeg, Canada, in the 1960s.

In August of 1965 in St. Boniface Hospital, Janet Reimer gave birth to two boys: Bruce and his identical twin, Brian, beautiful babies with upturned noses and small round mouths. Janet and her husband, Ron—young parents who had been married just the year before—were thrilled.

But several months later, the couple realized that their sons were having difficulty urinating, so they brought them to a pediatrician. Both boys were diagnosed with a condition called phimosis, in which the foreskin of the penis is so tight it can't be pulled back. The treatment was circumcision, and the boys were scheduled for surgery.

On the day the twins were to have their circumcisions, the pediatrician who usually performed them was out. Instead, a general practitioner named Dr. Jean-Marie Huot was asked to circumcise the twins. Bruce was taken back for surgery first. While operating on him, Dr. Huot decided to use an electrocautery knife for this procedure—a knife that uses an electrically heated blade to prevent excessive bleeding. Unfortunately, the blade malfunctioned, and Bruce's penis was burned beyond repair.

The parents were brought into a room to meet with the doctor, who told them the news. Janet was shocked and later recounted to *Rolling Stone* magazine, "It was like a little string. And it went right up to the base, up to his body." Over the next few days, the burnt tissue dried and broke away in pieces.

Janet and Ron were devastated, as any parents would be. What kind of life was Bruce going to have? They sought medical opinions from around the country, even flying to the Mayo Clinic in Rochester, Minnesota. Each doctor essentially told the family that surgically constructing a penis was too difficult and that they didn't have a great option.

Then one day, seven months after the accident, the parents saw a doctor on TV talking about gender. The confident and charismatic doctor turned out to be Dr. Money. The parents wrote him a letter, and to their surprise, he wrote back that he wanted to meet them. They soon found themselves traveling to Johns Hopkins University in Baltimore.

Money told the parents his theory that gender was determined entirely by the environment. He recommended that Bruce have his penis removed and a vagina surgically constructed in its stead. He then instructed the parents to raise Bruce as a girl named Brenda and to check in with Money annually. The parents took his advice, and Brenda underwent a surgical vaginoplasty to create a vagina.

The family began raising Brenda as a girl and flew to Baltimore periodically to meet with Money and his team. During these visits, he put the twins through "therapy" that he believed would help Brenda to identify as female. The twins would later tell journalists that these therapies were bizarre and traumatic. One of the twins recounted to journalist John Colapinto that the therapy involved "childhood sexual rehearsal play," in which Money would instruct Bruce to push his crotch against Brenda's buttocks. Dr. Money thought such experiences were vital for Brenda to develop a female gender identity.

At age thirteen, the parents were instructed to give Brenda estrogen pills so her body would take on a more female form. But by that time, she was depressed and suicidal. Every time her mother tried to put her in a dress, she would scream. Brenda later told journalists that though she didn't say it at the time, she constantly felt like a boy. While Money published in the academic literature that Brenda had settled comfortably into the female gender role, the reality was that she was constantly gender dysphoric and hated when anyone treated her like a girl. At one point, she told her parents she would take her own life if she needed to visit Dr. Money again.

While it can be difficult for cisgender people to think of their transcendent sense of their gender identity, Brenda perhaps offers a prime example of the difficult-to-put-into-words feelings that arise when a cisgender person is subjected to the type of experience transgender people experience. Brenda was, in a very real way, a cisgender person experiencing gender dysphoria.

Brenda's parents eventually told her about her past. At fifteen, Brenda transitioned back to living as male, renamed himself David, and started taking testosterone. Wanting to stop this from happening to other people, he went public with his story in a 1997 *Rolling Stone* article written by John Colapinto, which the journalist later expanded on in the book *As Nature Made Him: The Boy Who Was Raised as a Girl.* The article created a dramatic stir in the medical and scientific communities. Dr. Money had been telling the world for years that David's situation, published as the "John-Joan case," had definitively established that gender was entirely dictated by our environments. And it turned out to be a lie. Experts began to realize that gender was not 100 percent socially constructed, as Money had claimed. It was too late, however, to undo the damage already done to the Reimer family. David died from suicide at age thirty-eight.

In 2005, Columbia University psychologist Heino Meyer-Bahlburg published a comprehensive review of cases like David's. In reviewing the literature, he found seven cases of children with XY chromosomes who had traumatic loss of the penis during childhood and were subsequently raised as female. Of these, two were living with a male gender expression, four were living as females, and one was living as a female but expressed feelings of gender dysphoria. This heterogeneity raised some questions about the nature-versus-nurture question of gender identity, given that several of these individuals continued to live as female, as Money had predicted.

However, Dr. Meyer-Bahlburg expands on this, giving several reasons why some of these papers may have reported that these patients identified as female. Many of the people were still quite young at the time they were interviewed—most seemed to still be in their teens or twenties. It's possible that they were not yet open with others about their true feelings. In fact, after publication of the paper, one of the patients listed was mentioned in a *Globe and Mail* story, which explained that he was living as male, not female. Meyer-Bahlburg highlighted that it was often the case that these patients did not feel comfortable telling doctors or their parents how they truly felt, due to fear of how others would react. He even mentioned another case in which a person did not come out as male until both his parents had died, presumably worried about how they would have reacted while they were still alive. Reading this, I thought of the adult transgender people I've met who similarly didn't feel comfortable coming out as trans while their parents were alive to hear about it. I thought back to Susan, the trans woman who didn't come out until her sixties, and the deep sense of loss she felt related to missing so many decades of being her authentic self. In addition to this mourning, she also mourned how hiding who she truly was impacted her ability to have a deep authentic relationship with her parents. The colleague I met over coffee, who had recently moved to San Francisco, also explained that not being able to tell their parents about their gender-related experience meant that they never really got close to them— since their parents never got to know the real person they were.

While Meyer-Bahlburg's review complicated the David Reimer picture a bit, something seemed clear: there was some biological driving force impacting the thoughts and behaviors of these young people so that they did not universally grow up to identify as female, despite every effort to raise them in this way. But the question remained: Where did this come from?

TWIN STUDIES: SEPARATING GENES FROM ENVIRONMENT

Since David Reimer's death, scientists have accumulated a large body of evidence showing that there are strong biological determinants of our gender identities. One way that researchers examine the influence of environment versus genetics on the development of different conditions is through twin studies. In these studies, researchers look at people with a given trait (in this case transgender identity) who happen to be twins. Some of these twins will be monozygotic twins. That is, they share identical DNA and are sometimes referred to as identical twins.* Others will be dizygotic twins, those who have different DNA. They are sometimes referred to as fraternal twins. Generally, twins are raised in the same family and are thought to have similar environments, allowing researchers to look at whether genetics impact a certain variable, even when the environment is fairly constant. By looking at monozygotic and dizygotic twins, researchers can see if a condition has an innate biological basis that is encoded in our DNA.

Twin studies related to gender identity have suggested that the core of our gender identities has strong biological underpinnings. In 2012, a team of researchers published a study in the *Journal of Sexual Medicine.* The researchers were able to identify forty-four sets of twins in which one twin had what was at the time called "gender identity disorder," the prelude to the term *gender dysphoria.*† The authors of the study noted that among the

---

* David Reimer and his brother were identical, monozygotic twins. This is part of the reason Dr. Money was so interested in their case, as he believed they would offer the perfect experiment to show that social environment, not genetics, dictated gender identity.

† One problem with twin studies examining gender identity is that most used these outdated diagnoses that focused largely on gender role behavior rather than gender identity per se. A major limitation of these studies is that it's hard to know for sure that these people were transgender and not merely cisgender people with gender "atypical" interests and behaviors. Nonetheless, such studies do give us some interesting information about the biological basis of our gendered selves. Furthermore, twin studies that have looked specifically at transgender identities have had similar findings (e.g., Diamond, *International Journal of Transgenderism,* 2013).

twins of people with gender identity disorder that had identical DNA, 40 percent of these twins also met criteria. In contrast, among those with different DNA (dizygotic twins), none did. Thus, whether we are cisgender or transgender seemed to be deeply rooted in an innate biological factor: our genes.

Though one might expect 100 percent of the identical twins to be transgender, we need to keep in mind that people often conceal their gender identity from researchers due to fear of stigma. We've also learned over time that genetics are somewhat more complicated than DNA alone. Researchers have established that though twins may have identical DNA, this DNA is modified over time by "epigenetic factors" that change which genes are activated. Some researchers have theorized that these epigenetic changes may also influence gender identity. These complexities aside, the twin research provides one piece of the puzzle and strong evidence that our gender identities have some sort of innate biological underpinnings, despite the details not yet being fully clear.

DIFFERENCES OF SEXUAL DEVELOPMENT

Another piece of the puzzle comes from what scientists call "differences of sexual development" (sometimes called intersex conditions). These are conditions in which the various domains of sex don't all neatly align as "male" or "female"—the types that John Money studied prior to the David Reimer "experiment."

If you saw Belgian model Hanne Gaby Odiele in her *Vogue* photo shoots, with her piercing blue eyes, porcelain-doll features, and slicked-back blond hair, you would not know she has androgen insensitivity syndrome, a condition in which people with XY (i.e., "male") chromosomes do not respond to testosterone. While Odiele makes testosterone similar to other people with XY chromosomes, her cells do not have working receptors to respond to it. People with this condition by and large appear "female," though they have a shallow vaginal cavity, no uterus, and undescended testicles. Odiele, like most people with androgen insensitivity syndrome, identifies as female.

Cases such as Odiele's suggest that such testosterone receptors may be important in the development of our gender identities. In a 2005 review article that examined 156 people with complete androgen insensitivity syndrome, it appeared that all identified as female, with none pursuing masculinizing gender-affirming medical care. While some scientists have argued that these people tend to be raised as female due to the appearance of their external genitalia, and thus social factors may be responsible for the overwhelming majority having female gender identities, other experts have found this less convincing. Odiele, for example, told the *Guardian* in 2017 that she became aware of her condition at age seventeen. Unlike David Reimer, however, this did not impact her female gender identity. Though she has incorporated her intersex status into her identity and feels it has given her a unique perspective on gender, she continues to have a female gender identity and expression.

Another difference of sexual development that provides glimpses into the biology of gender identity is 5-alpha reductase 2 (5αR2) deficiency. For people who have XY (i.e., "male") chromosomes and this condition, their bodies experience a unique situation that essentially causes them to go from a "female" physical appearance before puberty to a "male" physical appearance once puberty begins.

The enzyme 5aR2 is responsible for converting testosterone into a related chemical called dihydrotestosterone, which plays an important role during fetal development in forming the genitals.

While there is some diversity in presentations at birth, most XY newborns with 5aR2 deficiency have either female-appearing genitalia or male-appearing genitalia that are not fully developed. Often the condition goes undiagnosed, as families and physicians presume these children have XX chromosomes and will have a female gender identity. Though such people generally have undescended testes, they tend to go unnoticed.

When people with this condition reach puberty, those testes start to make testosterone, and they undergo the general physical changes of testosterone puberty (while external genital formation for a fetus needs dihydrotestosterone, many of the physical changes of puberty are driven by unmodified testosterone). A 2005 review article found that among such people, around 60 percent change their gender expression from female to male around the time of puberty. While again, this could be related to how such people are socialized based on their physical appearance, it may also implicate sex hormones in gender identity.

The organization interACT aims to support and advocate for people with differences of sexual development (again, sometimes called intersex conditions). In December of 2022, I spent time with its communications director, Maddie Moran (*they/them* pronouns), and its legal and policy director, Sylvan Fraser (*they/them* pronouns). Maddie and Sylvan's perspectives on the interplay between gender identity and intersex conditions are important to highlight. While they agreed with the general framing I explain here about what intersex conditions may tell us about the origins of gender identity, they emphasized that intersex people have unique experiences of gender identity compared to most trans people who are not intersex. They also expressed frustration with the experiences of intersex people being used by people on both sides of the political aisle, without focusing on their unique needs. InterACT works to educate medical providers and the public on the experiences of people with differences of sexual development, and the organization is focused on the history of the medical profession performing surgical procedures on intersex infants prior to their being able to express their gender identities in their own words.

While surgeons sometimes argue that genital procedures are safer for infants than for older adolescents, interACT points to many of its members for whom their gender identity trajectory assumed by doctors did not match how they grew up to identify. Many are furious about the procedures done on them as infants. Maddie and Sylvan explained that though, for certain conditions, doctors can predict with 90 percent accuracy what people's gender identity may be in the future, irreversible surgery for the other 10 percent whose gender can't be predicted is of concern to them, particularly because the infants are too young to provide any kind of opinion. Despite the study I mentioned that found 100 percent of patients with complete androgen insensitivity syndrome identified as female, Maddie and Sylvan point out that there are people in their organization with the condition who identify as male, emphasizing that the medical literature often fails to represent their full community.

The medical profession in some ways seems to be slowly catching up with the perspectives of Maddie and Sylvan when it comes to giving young people more autonomy in decision-making. In 2022, doctors from Oregon wrote about a young patient with 5αR2 deficiency, the condition in which people are generally born with a "female" physical appearance but undergo a masculinizing testosterone puberty. Following that patient's lead, and borrowing from the approaches used in gender-affirming medical care for trans youth, they offered a puberty blocker, the same kind of medication Meredith used to pause puberty. This gave the patient more time to reflect and decide what was right for them in terms of what puberty they wanted to have.

In many ways, the people from interACT share the perspectives of those advocating for gender-affirming medical care for trans adolescents: don't make assumptions, and let people tell you their gender identities in their own words and in their own time. Let them make their own decisions about any medical or surgical interventions that relate to that. In both instances—gender-affirming care for trans people and intersex surgical considerations—advocates want people to get in-depth information about the risks, benefits, and potential side effects of interventions so that they can make the best decisions for themselves. But they both emphasize that individual people are the experts on their own highly personal gender identities, which may or may not align with doctors' or society's predictions.

THE GUINEA PIG AND RHESUS CHRONICLES: WHAT NON-HUMAN ANIMALS CAN TELL US ABOUT GENDER

Another line of scientific research that gives us insight into the biological basis of our, and our children's, gender identities, involves an unexpected animal: the guinea pig. Around the same time that John Money was counseling the Reimers about how to raise their child, researchers from the University of Kansas published a landmark study. In their 1959 paper in the journal *Endocrinology*, Charles Phoenix and his colleagues wrote about what happened when they injected pregnant guinea pigs with testosterone. It was a strange experiment that nonetheless had a dramatic impact on our understanding of hormones and brain development.

The XX offspring of pregnant guinea pigs injected with testosterone had masculine appearing genitalia. However, the researchers noticed that it wasn't just their anatomy that changed—their behavior was also different. These XX guinea pigs started to exhibit "male" guinea pig behavior—for example, mounting other guinea pigs. Additionally, most XX guinea pigs, when given the ovarian hormones estradiol and progesterone, will go into a position called lordosis, in which they arch their back in preparation for sexual intercourse. However, the guinea pigs that were treated with testosterone in utero did not.

One could have assumed that these guinea pigs had different behaviors because they looked different (their genitals were different, so many other guinea pigs treated them more like boys, impacting their behavior)—an argument similar to what some say about the differences of sexual development literature and gender identity. But Phoenix and his colleagues ran experiments that argued against this. They found that when the pregnant guinea pigs were treated with lower doses of testosterone, their genitalia did not masculinize—they looked like other XX guinea pigs. However, they still exhibited the more "male-like" behavior. And this behavior was long-lasting. It seemed that prenatal hormonal milieu had a dramatic organizing effect on the brain, setting a foundation that would be there for life.

These researchers realized that their findings might have important implications beyond rodents and for that reason became interested in working with animals that were more closely related to humans: rhesus monkeys.

Rhesus monkeys are interesting because researchers can study behaviors beyond just sexual ones like lordosis and mounting.* For example, XY monkeys make distinct vocalizations, engage more in rough-and-tumble play, and are more likely to initiate play. In contrast, XX monkeys have their own distinct vocalizations and tend to show a greater interest in infants.

Before I go into these experiments, it's worth noting that there are examples of gender diversity without any external manipulation among nonhuman primates. In his book *Different*, primatologist Frans de Waal writes about a chimpanzee named Donna. Donna, though she had a female sex according to de Waal, had behaviors more typical of male monkeys. She would sit poised like other male monkeys, and when the male monkeys started to hoot and "bluff around," she would join in and charge by their sides. She was the only monkey designated female at birth who would make the vocalizations similar to those of adult males, albeit hers were higher pitched. Her sex-atypical behaviors were not, however, sexual in nature. She never sought sexual contact with other female-sex chimps. In an example of chimpanzees outperforming humans, de Waal

---

* It's worth noting that for many years people hypothesized that in utero exposure to testosterone was a major determinant of sexual orientation. This theory never played out with definitive convincing evidence.

explained that the other chimpanzees accepted Donna and her gender diversity: "It was just part of who [Donna] was, and . . . the other apes didn't seem to mind. [Donna] had a happy-go-lucky attitude and got along with everyone." As with humans, it appeared that gender identity and expression were a separate phenomenon from sexual orientation, though the chimpanzees did a better job of being accepting.

Let's go back to the in utero rhesus experiments. Through the painstaking process of injecting pregnant rhesus monkeys with testosterone, then raising the offspring, researchers were able to confirm the guinea pig findings in a species more closely related to humans. The results were apparent from the first two testosterone-exposed XX monkeys that the researchers reported on. These monkeys were more likely than XX monkeys without fetal testosterone exposure to engage in rough-and-tumble play, and they withdrew less from the approaches of other animals, while also trying to mount the other monkeys more often.

In the late 1980s, researchers published a study looking at the timing of testosterone treatment in pregnancy and outcomes among the monkey offspring. They found that testosterone treatment early in pregnancy masculinized the genitals but did not increase rough-and-tumble play. On the other hand, testosterone treatment late in pregnancy did not masculinize the genitals but did increase rough-and-tumble play.

This finding created an interesting hypothesis for the development of transgender identities. It made it clear that the genitals are formed early in development, whereas the hormone-sensitive aspects of brain development come later. It set up the possibility that for transgender people, the hormone milieu in the uterus may have changed over the course of pregnancy. For example, a "male hormone milieu" with more testosterone may be present early, resulting in the formation of the penis, but a "female hormone milieu" with more estrogen may then be present later, resulting in a more "female" brain.

Such a theory of course is nearly impossible to study in humans, and we can't ask guinea pigs and monkeys to speak with us about the complexities of their gender identities. However, these early studies did establish what scientists call the "organizational hypothesis," suggesting that prenatal factors have long-lasting impacts on our behaviors, and potentially our identities.[*]

It's difficult to know for sure, but the research seems to suggest that these factors may be what drive our difficult-to-put-into-words transcendent senses of our gender identities, upon which we build our identities throughout our lives.

MODERN GENDER SCIENCE

With the advent of more sophisticated scientific tools, researchers have brought the study of the biological basis of gender identity into the twenty-first century. In 2019, an

---

[*] One of the researchers who conducted these experiments was Milton Diamond. Diamond was often in intellectual disagreement with John Money and for years put out advertisements in psychiatry journals trying to find the mental health professionals who took over caring for David Reimer after John Money was no longer caring for him. Diamond ended up finding David and publishing the 1997 long-term follow-up paper that revealed Dr. Money's John-Joan experiment had failed (Diamond and Sigmundson, *Archives of Pediatrics & Adolescent Medicine*, 1997).

international team of researchers sequenced the genomes of thirteen transgender men and seventeen transgender women. Using gene sequencing and statistical strategies, they were able to identify several differences in the DNA that encodes proteins important in estrogen signaling pathways among the transgender study participants, again implicating hormones in the development of gender identity. Though they didn't identify a single "transgender gene," they provided additional evidence for an innate biological basis of our gender identities.

Other researchers have utilized neuroimaging techniques to noninvasively compare the brains of cisgender and transgender people. Results have been somewhat conflicting, and scientists have mixed feelings about how meaningful such neuroimaging studies are. Older neuroimaging studies would take crude measurements of different brain regions to try to see if, on average, trans people's brains looked more like others of their same gender identity or others of their same sex assigned at birth. Findings from these studies have been inconsistent at best. Even if they were consistent, many neuroscientists point out that crude measurements such as the average volume of a brain region aren't particularly informative, with some even comparing it to phrenology—the old pseudoscientific practice of measuring the shape and size of someone's skull to predict things such as intelligence. The brain is a complex network of neurons wired together into circuits, and the way the neurons talk to one another is probably more important than the size of a given part of the brain.

Some scientists have moved beyond measuring the sizes of brain regions into the realm of "functional neuroimaging" studies—those that look at how different brain regions become more active during specific tasks. These functional studies are often considered more informative than structural studies. One study looked at the brains of people while smelling chemicals that are known to create different patterns of brain activation among cisgender men and women (so-called human phero-mones). They found that results for trans people were some-where in between those for cisgender men and women. A 2021 review of all the different neuroimaging studies on sexual ori-entation and gender identity found countless different ways in which researchers have used various neuroimaging techniques to try to understand the connections between the brain and gender identity, but the results varied dramatically, and the best conclusion seemed to be that gender identity is too complex to boil down to a single neuroimaging measure. Again, given the complexity of gender identity, this isn't particularly surprising. To this date, there is no imaging technique that can tell whether someone is cisgender, transgender, or any other gender identity.

THE SEARCH FOR THE BIOLOGICAL BASIS OF GENDER IDENTITY: TO WHAT END?

Overall, a large body of research shows that gender identity has a strong biological basis. At the same time, we're far from identifying a single gene or brain region that determines one's gender identity. And that's perhaps not surprising. As we've seen, gender identity is a complex multidimensional construct that involves so many facets of ourselves. Nonetheless, I find myself reflecting on this literature and finding it hard not to conclude that our foundational gender identity is based on early innate biological factors. While we build upon this foundation and decorate it with life experience and language, the foundation itself seems to be there from the get-go and to stay with us for life.

It's also hard to reflect on this research and not ask ourselves, "Why are we doing this?" What motivates us to study the biological basis of gender identity? Some, including the authors of the whole exome genetic study, argue that if we find a biological basis of transgender identity, people will respect trans people more and it will be easier to protect their civil rights.

Others have pointed out that this research could just as easily be weaponized in the opposite direction. Does this tireless search for what "causes" someone to be transgender imply that being transgender is a pathology, something that needs to be fixed? Why are we taking a disease-model approach to studying something that's not a disease, but rather a normal aspect of human diversity? If we were to identify a "transgender gene," would that information one day be used to out people against their will by studying their genomes? Would it be used in embryo screenings so parents could avoid having transgender children, leading to a new eugenics?

It turns out the same debates were had around research into what determines someone's sexual orientation. Similar genetic studies were done to try to identify a "gay gene."* But

---

* Interestingly, these studies have suggested that male homosexuality may be linked to the X chromosome. A variation in one part of the X chromosome is thought to increase the likelihood of women with such DNA giving birth, while it results in male offspring being gay. The thought is that this balancing effect of increased reproductive potential for XX people with the gene and decreased reproductive potential for XY people with the gene balance each other out, so that there is a steady small proportion of gay men in the population.

we've never identified a clear-cut gene or brain region that "causes" homosexuality. Despite this, public perception of gay people and protection of their civil rights have dramatically improved over the past few decades. But this improvement wasn't driven primarily by figuring out the biological basis of sexual orientation. It largely came from more people coming out of the closet.

To learn more about this, I reached out to Evan Wolfson, a lawyer and LGBTQ civil rights advocate who created the organization Freedom to Marry, which fought for marriage equality prior to the organization's being dissolved after gay marriage became protected nationwide.

He explained to me that the growing notion that gay people are "born that way" likely played a role for some people when it came to gay civil rights. He reflected on how he would ask people when they first realized they were straight, which helped them realize that sexual orientation wasn't a choice for them. You could, of course, ask people similar questions about their gender identity. But he also pointed out that there were major historical phenomena that resulted in more gay people coming out of the closet, and that as more Americans knew gay people who were impacted by antigay politics, public opinion shifted.

One major historical event was World War II. The war brought America's young men from around the country and put them together in large gateway cities like San Francisco and New York. Gay men from more rural areas who would never have met a gay person came to meet other gay people either through the military or the more open gay communities in these big cities. AIDS represented another major historical event, as the deadly disease pushed more people to come out of the closet and increased urgency for gay people to be recognized and supported.

As gay people became more visible, straight people realized that gay people were either their loved ones, or the loved ones of other people who were important to them. Over time, people found antigay legislation unacceptable, and we saw major advances in gay rights.

Evan pointed out that the American Psychiatric Association removed homosexuality from the *DSM* in 1973, presumably a major piece of "biological" evidence for many Americans. He went on to highlight that it didn't change things right away. It took more time and more people coming out for people to recognize the common humanity, shared values, and empathy that ultimately pushed gay rights forward.

Perhaps what's more important than research on where gender identity comes from is research on how we can best support transgender people and help them thrive. As Dallas Ducar, CEO of Transhealth, a health center entirely dedicated to serving the trans community across New England, told me, "At the end of the day, it doesn't matter why someone is trans. What matters is how we can help trans people be happy and healthy." It's important that we not get lost in complex scientific arguments and lose sight of the fact that there are over 1 million transgender people in the United States, and that each is an individual human being deserving of love and respect. While the research on the biological basis of our gender identities is helpful in understanding ourselves and how the foundations of our gender identities form, we should provide humans with dignity and respect regardless.

Some of the issues that come up in searching for a "cause" of transgender identities become clearer when we take a look at past flawed research that tried to suggest that diverse gender identities were a result of pathological environments and, in particular, bad parenting. We'll explore that history in the next chapter.

4

It's Always the Mom

The Pseudoscience of Blaming Parents and Social Environments

Despite the strong evidence that transness has an innate biological basis, I still find that people (particularly in the media) are constantly looking for social or environmental "causes" of being transgender. It's often the case that this search starts with looking at parents. Parents of trans youth often find themselves being "blamed" for their kids being transgender. It's wrong because it falsely implies that there's any evidence that parents can control their child's gender identity. It's also wrong because it implies that being trans is a bad outcome—something to be avoided—and thus that "blame" is even a valid concept. Sadly, much of this parent-blaming phenomenon has its roots in the history of psychiatry, which has a long sordid past of attributing innate biological phenomena (gender identity, autism, and even schizophrenia) to parenting styles.

In June of 2021, I met with Katie and her family to talk about their experience of Katie coming out as transgender in a conservative Southern state. Katie was eighteen years old and grew up in a small town in Tennessee. When I first met her, she was sitting at her family's dining room table, leaning so far forward it seemed as if she would curl up into herself. As she moved her wavy blond hair away from her face, her kind brown eyes revealed a hint of sadness. But after a few minutes, once it became clear that I accepted her for who she was (I called her Katie and used *she/her* pronouns), her posture corrected, and she became vibrant and confident. The sadness in her eyes evaporated into joy, and a new touch of sass accompanied the Southern twang in her voice. We spoke more about her life, and Katie and her mom told me that Katie is a nationally renowned fencer, beloved by her friends and her coach in particular, who, by all accounts, is quick to tell everyone she's the most talented athlete he has ever worked with.

Katie's mom, Jillian, is a data scientist, and her dad, Mark, is an executive at a software company. Katie has a younger brother, Kevin, whom she adores. I'm always skeptical when kids say they don't fight with their siblings, so I pushed the question a little: "You two *never* fight?" Katie laughed and let me know that they fight about small things, like the TV remote, but that he truly is one of the most important people in her life. He had one of the best reactions when she came out as transgender: he didn't make a big deal about it. He still just saw her as the sibling he loved (and from whom he would always steal the remote when she went to the bathroom). Katie's mom shared that Kevin suffers from a rare collagen disease, which required him to be in and out of the hospital for many years when he was younger, putting a strain on the family. He's now healthy and doing well, but Katie is still very protective of him.

One of the most striking things about their family is how open they are. "People sometimes think we're weird because we don't fight, but really we just have a philosophy to always say what we think, so disagreements get resolved fast," Jillian explained.

Even so, for years there was something Katie felt she couldn't put on the table: she didn't really feel like a boy. She spent over a decade afraid that if she told her parents or anyone at school, she would be bullied or rejected. And she had good reason. When she was in elementary school, she tried to hold her friend Charles's hand in the lunch line. She thought it was a nice way to show that she cared about him. But her mother was called into the principal's office the following day and told that Charles's family "doesn't put up with that homosexual stuff" and that Katie wasn't to be friends with Charles or to go anywhere near him. The message was clear: conform, or you'll be in big trouble.

As Katie put it, "I went so far in the closet I was in Narnia."

It's sadly a common experience for people to hide or sacrifice who they are in order to fit in, avoid social ostracism, and establish connection. Humans are hardwired to want to affiliate with others. It can be easy to overlook the potential pitfalls of this. Dr. Brené Brown explains it well when she discusses the difference between "fitting in" and "belonging." Under her framework, *fitting in* means being like others to be accepted, whereas *belonging* means showing up and saying, "This is who I am. I hope we can make a connection." This second approach allows for greater self-confidence, less shame, and deeper, more genuine connection. Sadly, many trans kids like Katie aren't given that option.

Katie has a vivid memory of going to Spirit Halloween with her mom and brother in fourth grade. She remembers walking through the aisles seeing Godzilla heads, vampire fangs, and creepy clown costumes. None of them felt right for her, and if anything, they made her feel scared. "Seriously—what's with that clown from *It*? I get the heebie-jeebies just thinking about him." Moving through the aisles, she looked down at her feet and hastened past the *Scream* masks. When she looked up again, she saw a bright orange tutu hanging at the end of the next aisle. She let out a small gasp. It was perfect. She called her mom over to show her. Katie beamed in the car on the way home, the Spirit Halloween bag on her lap overflowing with the tutu and a green Morphsuit (one of those tight bodysuits that covers the whole body).

When she got home, she ran up the stairs to her room to change into her outfit and get ready for a school Halloween party that night. But as she stood in her bedroom doorway, her dad saw her and yelled, "Whoa, whoa, you can't wear that! People will think you're trying to be a girl!" Katie's heart sank into her stomach. It was one of her earliest and most intense experiences of gender threat, and a strong message that the expectation was to "fit in" not "belong," even within her own family. She looked at her dad for a second, then looked away. She pulled the tutu down, kicked it off her shoes, and didn't say another word about it. She went to the party in just the Morphsuit, which hid the tears rolling down her bright red cheeks. From that moment on, she vowed to present herself as being as masculine as possible, forcing her voice to sound deeper and throwing herself into sports that people would think were manly, including football and baseball. Over time, she developed the slumped posture I noticed when I first met her, a physical manifestation of her attempts to disappear from public sight. She also became depressed.

In her quest to appear masculine, Katie did find one sport she loved: fencing. For years, Katie's fencing coach would comment to her mother that Katie had all the skills needed to be the best fencer on the team, but something held her back, and she had never won a match. He always felt she was hiding something, and that whatever it was had made her deeply sad.

At seventeen, Katie finally came out as transgender. To her surprise, her friends and parents accepted her. It was rocky with her parents at first, but they came around quickly. Katie's dad doesn't remember the tutu incident and regrets the way he made his daughter feel as a child. With her secret revealed, Katie's depression improved and so did her fencing. Her mother told me that with the emotional weight off Katie's shoulders, she started to win every fencing match (she was still competing on the boys' team). Her coach was thrilled to see her happy and reaping the rewards of her athletic skill. Katie's quick to point out that coming out helped her depression dramatically, but she's still impacted by the years she spent closeted and by seeing attacks on trans people in the media.

While Katie's friends and family handled her news well, not everyone was pleased. Some aunts and uncles stopped talking to Katie and her parents. Her parents were inundated with questions about what they did to make Katie transgender. Jillian was flooded with accusations that her child's transgender identity was her "fault." The time-honored American tradition of parent blaming had begun.

One of Katie's therapists told Jillian that Katie probably became transgender because her mother spent so much time taking care of Kevin when he was in and out of the hospital. The therapist refused to talk to Katie about her gender identity, telling her she would identify as a boy again if they just continued to work on her depression. Not surprisingly, given how invalidating that approach is, Katie does not think highly of this therapist and no longer sees him. She's quick to point out, "He didn't get my depression any better either."

When Jillian told one of her best friends that Katie had come out as transgender, her friend's first question was "Do you think it was because of that porn thing?"

When Katie was in elementary school, she and a few classmates got in trouble for searching for *hooters* on a school computer while working on a project about owls. With the inadvertent Google search, they fell down an internet rabbit hole. Jillian's friend was convinced that poor maternal oversight had made Katie transgender. Jillian was taken aback. How was school computer use her fault? And why would googling *hooters* make someone transgender? But Jillian was confused about Katie's gender identity, too. Instead of questioning her friend or fighting with her, Jillian simply withdrew from the relationship and became more depressed herself.

Soon after that, Jillian's neighbor Mark called the house and asked if her kids would help him move some boxes. Wanting to avoid any uncomfortable situations, Jillian told Mark that the kids would be happy to, but that he should know Katie had recently come out as transgender and was now wearing dresses. Mark snapped back, "How could you let your child do that?" He then declined the help and decided to move the boxes himself. At every turn, Jillian felt judged. It seemed everyone thought that Katie's gender identity was a result of bad parenting and that Jillian was wrong to support her.

Of course, this kind of maternal blame is not unique to questions of gender identity. As a society we have a strong tendency to blame mothers for anything going on with their children, even when the "problem" isn't a real problem, as in Katie's case.

When children have meltdowns in grocery stores and airplanes, we always hear people ask, "What is wrong with those parents?" It's rarely someone's first instinct to consider that the child's outburst is from biologically determined ADHD, a medication side effect, or a medical condition. Our default is to point fingers at the parents, and usually the mother.

But why do we always blame moms like Jillian when it comes to a child's mental health or behavior? Psychiatry has likely played a major role here. The field has historically blamed mothers for a wide range of biologically based conditions* in their children, from schizophrenia to autism spectrum disorder—to, of course, being transgender.

---

* I intentionally use the word *conditions* here to highlight that phenomena like gender diversity and autistic traits are often inappropriately pathologized when they are not "issues" but rather healthy variations of the human experience.

THE ORIGIN OF MOTHER BLAMING

Our tendency to blame moms for mental health problems can be traced back to the founder of psychoanalysis: Austrian physician Sigmund Freud. Many of Freud's foundational theories, presented in the early 1900s, involve how early childhood experiences—particularly relationships with parents—can create future psychopathology. You've probably heard of the Oedipus complex, Freud's theory that a child's desire to have sex with or murder their parents determines that child's later mental health. With an emphasis on social and environmental factors—in particular, parenting—as causes of mental illness, Freud placed nurture over nature. His underlying argument was that environmental trauma could be overcome through talk therapy, and his theories soon became gospel among psychiatrists.

Early in my medical training, a senior psychiatrist told me about a young boy who came to see him weekly for therapy. In every session, the patient would take a toy sword from the corner of the office and pretend to stab the doctor. He would play along and fall to the floor screaming, *"No!"*

The psychiatrist told me that this could be conceptualized as being due to the boy's mother divorcing his father, so the boy never experienced what Freud described as "an Oedipal defeat," in which a child learns that he can't have a romantic relationship with his mother because of his father. The psychiatrist theorized that this was why the child had become aggressive. To this day, I find it more convincing that the boy just thought having a toy sword in a doctor's office was weird and fun. He was also probably annoyed that he had to spend time with a child psychiatrist instead of his friends. But the case highlights how pervasive Freud's sometimes bizarre theories continue to be and how they shape the ways the mental health field thinks about parents.

Following World War II, Freud's ideas were a welcome contrast to the Nazis' focus on nature over nurture and their eugenicist philosophies. Unfortunately, this meant more mom blaming. Frieda Fromm-Reichmann, an Orthodox Jewish German psychiatrist who fled to the United States during World War II, became one of the most prominent psychiatrists to blame mothers for their children's mental illness. Dr. Fromm-Reichmann specialized in the treatment of schizophrenia, a condition that impacts a little under 1 percent of the U.S. population and in which people lose touch with reality, often become paranoid, and may start hearing voices that aren't there.

Today, we know that schizophrenia has a strong innate biological basis, requires medication for treatment, and does not get better with talk therapy alone. But Dr. Fromm-Reichmann was a firm believer in psychoanalysis and in the "environmental" causes of mental and even physical illness. She was so sold on these theories that she thought her husband's tuberculosis infection was a manifestation of psychological distress from their tense romantic relationship (it wasn't, of course—tuberculosis is caused by a bacterium).

In 1948, she famously proposed in a journal article that schizophrenia was a result of poor mothering: "The schizophrenic is painfully distrustful and resentful of other people, due to the severe early warp and rejection he encountered in important people of his infancy and childhood, as a rule, mainly in a schizophrenogenic mother." The idea that mothers were responsible for their children's schizophrenia predominated until the 1970s, when American neuroscientist Seymour Kety published a seminal paper showing that children of mothers with schizophrenia who were raised by adoptive parents developed schizophrenia at the same rate as those who were raised by their biological mothers. Though the precise cause remains elusive, the broad scientific consensus is that schizophrenia is a biologically based condition and strongly determined by genetics, not by bad mothering. And talk therapy does not make the brain-based condition go away.

In my psychiatry residency, I treated an elderly woman with schizophrenia in the hospital psychiatry unit. When Ellen was taking medications and doing well, she would keep her gray hair in a neat ponytail, carrying her frail five-foot, three-inch frame with dignity. She often walked around the unit asking the other patients if she could bring them coffee. She ended every conversation with me by saying, "Thank you, Doctor," revealing her kindness and the value she placed on respect.

But even on her medication, she firmly believed that the FBI was following her everywhere she went and raping her. She heard their voices tell her that if she took her medications, they would kill her. Because of this, she would stop taking the medications every time she left the hospital and would within weeks be back in the emergency room screaming and spitting at the doctors, unable to deal with the horrible cacophony in her head. I later learned that she had been in this vicious cycle for decades.

She luckily had an extraordinarily supportive family. Ellen developed her symptoms in her twenties, and her mother, who has since passed away, dedicated her life to finding Ellen when she ran away and trying to convince her to come home and take her medications. But Ellen, afraid that the FBI would hurt her family, always refused. To this day, her brothers desperately try to look after her. They send her money and offer her places to live, but she turns them down, consumed with guilt that the FBI will do something to hurt the family that has been so good to her. The idea that these devoted family members, burdened with this unimaginable pain, are somehow to blame for Ellen's illness is infuriating and preposterous. Psychiatry has thankfully moved past this cruel theory—at least when it comes to schizophrenia.

THE REFRIGERATOR MOTHER: IS AUTISM YOUR MOM'S FAULT?

Psychiatry and society's tendencies toward parent blaming go far beyond schizophrenia. Perhaps one of the most famous examples lies in the historical descriptions of autism spectrum disorder.* In 1943, around the time Dr. Fromm-Reichmann was blaming mothers for their children's schizophrenia, Austrian psychiatrist Leo Kanner at Johns Hopkins University described a condition he called early infantile autism, a precursor to today's diagnosis of autism spectrum disorder. Though the diagnostic criteria for this condition have evolved over the years, they generally include difficulties with social skills and intense obsessional interests. In addition, many people with the condition demonstrate incredibly strong attention to detail.

---

* There are also some interesting parallels with gender identity here in that autism is often inappropriately pathologized.

As a psychiatry resident, I met Mary, a fifteen-year-old girl with autism. With her curly red hair and freckles, her parents often compared her to Aileen Quinn, the star of the movie *Annie*, whom Mary admires. Her symptoms of autism were classic. She was obsessed with trains and could tell you precisely how their engines work. She loved her family but was less interested in making friends, and she found social situations confusing. She rarely made eye contact and didn't always understand why people took offense when she said something that was true. ("But she does have acne—why did I get in trouble for saying that? I'm sure she was aware. I thought my advice to try other skin-care options was helpful.") Mary was also brilliant and already taking advanced college math classes. Her autism allowed her to focus in a way that people without autism rarely can. Her mother, a fifth-grade teacher, and her father, a social worker, were warm and supportive. They had exceptionally affectionate interpersonal styles and had gone above and beyond to support their daughter.

Kanner primarily believed that autism was innate, but he noted that the mothers of children with autism spectrum disorder often seemed cold and intellectual. He coined a special phrase for them: "refrigerator mothers." In retrospect, his observations were probably because the majority of his patients were the children of parents who worked at his university. These parents were, therefore, much more "intellectual" than most people and understandably approached Kanner with the professional demeanor they showed coworkers. Given that autism has a strong genetic component, some of the parents may also have exhibited autistic traits themselves, which they passed on through genetics rather than through their approach to childcare.

A few decades later, in the 1960s and 1970s, University of Chicago psychologist Bruno Bettelheim took particular interest in the notion of the refrigerator mother and ultimately declared that autism was not a result of biology at all but of cold, distant mothers. Bettelheim, a Holocaust survivor held in Nazi concentration camps for ten months prior to fleeing from Vienna to the United States, went so far as to compare these mothers to the Nazi guards in concentration camps. The caricatures he created could not be more different from Mary's parents. Bettelheim was widely known for advocating "parentectomy"—that is, cutting children off from their parents by placing them in a residential treatment facility, such as his own program, the Orthogenic School.* Due to his charismatic personality, Bettelheim was often quoted in the media, and his ideas about autism became widespread.

Around the time that Bettelheim's ideas were gaining traction in the United States, recently married psychologist Bernard Rimland became a father. His child, Mark, was difficult to manage. Bernard and his wife, Gloria Belle Alf, struggled with the fact that their child wasn't affectionate toward them in the ways they had hoped. He also spoke with unusually repetitive speech. Concerned, Bernard started poring over old psychology textbooks and came across autism. A pediatrician later confirmed

---

* In telling this story, I'm reminded of recent actions by Governor Greg Abbott of Texas, who labeled the affirmation of trans children "child abuse" and directed the state's child protective services to investigate families. Many subsequently fled the state to avoid having their children taken away from them.

that Mark met criteria for the diagnosis. Rimland continued studying the condition and learned about the predominant theory that autism was caused by cold, distant mothers.

This made no sense to him: Gloria was so warm and loving. Over time, Rimland developed a near-obsessional interest in the field and found disturbing flaws in the evidence behind the refrigerator mother theory. In 1964, he published the book *Infantile Autism: The Syndrome and Its Implications for a Neural Theory of Behavior*, in which he proposed a return to the theory that the condition was innate and biologically based. In the years that followed, the evidence convincingly showed that autism had a strong biological basis. Most notably, in a 1977 study, Susan Folstein and Michael Rutter examined identical twins (those with the same genes) and fraternal twins (those with different genes) and found that identical twins were far more likely to both have autism than fraternal twins. As with schizophrenia, the parents of these children were vindicated. The parallels between Gloria and Bernard's experiences and those of Katie's parents are difficult to ignore: the parents were pathologized by pseudoscientific theories that dominated popular knowledge despite waning scientific support.

The refrigerator mother theory has since been broadly discredited, and scientists continue to add to our understanding of the biological basis for autism. But as Dr. Fred Volkmar, professor of child psychiatry at the Yale Child Study Center and editor in chief of the influential *Journal of Autism and Developmental Disorders*, told me, "It took the profession decades to realize that autism was brain based and strongly genetic."

One would think psychiatrists would have learned from their colleagues and their own mistakes. But theories persist that parents and social factors are the primary determinants of our psychology, even in circumstances in which biological data suggest otherwise.

BLAMING MOTHERS FOR GENDER DIVERSITY

Though blaming moms for their kids' autism fell out of favor by the 1970s, psychiatrists and psychologists continued to argue that parents made their children transgender well into the 1990s. A select few continue to push this pseudoscientific narrative today. Perhaps one of the most famous researchers to theorize about environmental causes of being transgender was UCLA psychiatrist Dr. Robert Stoller. In his 1975 book, *Sex and Gender*, he proposed the theory of "blissful symbiosis." His idea was that the moms of transgender girls were too involved with their children. As a result, he posited, "The child never quite learned where [her] mother left off and [she] began."

Stoller ultimately tested this hypothesis by running a study in which he examined how much time the mothers of transgender children spent with their kids compared to the mothers of cisgender children. His study ended up finding that the mothers of transgender girls actually spent *less* time with their kids than the mothers of cisgender children, disproving his blissful symbiosis theory.

Researchers later proposed the exact opposite theory: perhaps children become transgender because their mothers are too distant and unavailable. In their 1995 book, *Gender Identity Disorder and Psychosexual Problems in Children and Adolescents*, Canadian researchers Kenneth Zucker and Susan Bradley wrote about a child who they believed became transgender because her mother was depressed and withdrawn while her own mother, the child's grandmother, was ill: "[The mother] began to retreat to her bedroom for time alone and recalled that it was at this point that her son began to play with dolls extensively in his room." They downplayed that the child may already have been drawn to playing with dolls and would have done so regardless of her mother's depression and withdrawal. Gender diversity was either caused by too much maternal involvement or too little—there was no way mothers could win.

In addition to studying whether moms were too close or too distant from their transgender kids, researchers also asked whether such mothers were generally "mentally ill." In 1991, two researchers from St. Luke's Roosevelt Hospital Center in New York City set out to formally examine this theory. They recruited moms of transgender and cisgender children and used scales to gauge the degree to which they suffered from depression and another mental health condition called borderline personality disorder. People with borderline personality disorder experience their emotions very intensely and have trouble coping with them; they also tend to struggle with being very sensitive to interpersonal rejection. The disorder has been dramatized in movies, including by Winona Ryder's character, Susanna, in *Girl, Interrupted.*

The researchers found that the mothers of transgender children scored higher on both scales. For the borderline personality disorder scale, the mothers of transgender children scored higher on a particular measure of "interpersonal sensitivity." According to this line of reasoning, these kids must have become transgender because their parents were mentally ill—or just sensitive.

But Meredith's mom, Suzanne, the professor I met at her home in New England, had a different interpretation: "If I ever seemed depressed or interpersonally sensitive, it's because people around us were pathologizing my child. Those things came after I knew Meredith was transgender, not before." Though the authors of the study claim that these mothers' mental health difficulties "usually predated the onset of consolidated gender identity disorder," their mental health problems were only measured and recorded after they came to gender clinics, and the small sample size of sixteen mothers of transgender girls makes the study too small to produce convincing conclusions regardless.

Another study conducted by Zucker and Bradley appears to contradict their earlier conclusions and to show that mental health difficulties experienced by mothers of transgender children had been driven by the way other people reacted to their children. Zucker and Bradley looked at how many of the mothers of "girls with gender identity disorder" who were evaluated in their clinic had required psychiatric hospitalization. Of the four who had a history of hospitalization, two were admitted after Zucker and Bradley's team assessed and, given their theories, likely pathologized their children.

It's hard to read the literature on transgender children and not view it as hostile toward mothers. In a 1988 paper, a psychiatrist named Leslie Lothstein went so far as to use a single case to suggest that being transgender is a result of mothers being angry and man hating. He wrote about a girl who had, he believed, become transgender because she overheard her mother deliver "antimale speeches" to her feminist discussion group. Lothstein was also puzzled by the fact that the girl's mother was incensed by her husband's pathologizing of their child's gender identity and threatened to leave the marriage if he continued to do so. There was no acknowledgment that a mother may justifiably be upset with her husband for unnecessarily calling their child mentally ill.

Over and over, researchers failed to establish that parental mental illness makes kids transgender. So they looked to whether it wasn't mental illness of the mother per se, but rather that these moms didn't place enough limits around gender diverse behaviors. We can call this the "pushover mother" theory. In 1991, Zucker and his team studied the degree to which mothers of transgender girls and cisgender boys discouraged feminine behavior from their kids. They found that the moms of the transgender girls were less likely to discourage feminine behavior.

I chatted with Meredith's mother about this soon after I spoke with her about the study of whether these moms were depressed with borderline personality disorder traits. She raised an eyebrow and said, "You try tearing a doll away from a five-year-old girl who desperately wants to play with it and see how that goes for you." Meredith chimed in from the next room, "Don't try to take my Xbox either!"

This idea of trying to force your child into a gender box is reminiscent of the carpenter approach to parenting, described by University of California, Berkeley, professor of psychology Dr. Alison Gopnik. In her 2016 book on the topic, she explains that many parents attempt to take on this so-called carpenter role to parenting—trying to mold their children into what the parents think they should be. She cautions that this approach can lead young people to feel tense, anxious, and unhappy, as they're unable to follow their natural childhood instincts of exploration and express their authentic selves. She advocates instead for a "gardener" approach, in which parents allow their children to explore their natural instincts, while providing nurture and protection, but not forced molding.

Dr. Fred Volkmar, the autism expert from Yale who spoke with me about the refrigerator mother theory, explained that autism researchers struggled for years to realize that not everything is about how parents impact their kids. The refrigerator mother had a powerful foothold for years. It wasn't until recently that people started to realize what in retrospect is obvious: children also impact their parents, as do societal attacks on people's children. If your child is struggling with autism, or with the stigma of people trying to pathologize the child's gender identity, you as a parent are going to be affected, too.

BEYOND MOMS: THE DESPERATE SEARCH FOR ALTERNATIVE CAUSES OF GENDER DIVERSITY

My hope is that understanding this history of parent blaming, and its flawed theoretical and scientific underpinnings, will help people fight the urge to attack the parents of trans kids and understand the dramatic toll it takes on parents when society at large seems to have it out for their kid. But I also want to focus in on the kids and how other damaging theories about what causes transness have propagated harm. Some of the non-parent-related theories around psychological causes of gender diversity are even more unusual than those blaming parents.

In *Sex and Gender*, Dr. Stoller noted that children who were assigned male at birth and identified as female "often ha[d] pretty faces, with fine hair, lovely complexions, graceful movements, and—especially—big, piercing, liquid eyes." Based on this observation, he came up with another theory: maybe transgender girls become transgender because they are so cute that everyone (not just their moms) treats them like girls, which makes them identify as female.

In 1993, Zucker and Bradley set out to test this hypothesis about transgender girls being very cute. They took headshots of seventeen children assigned male at birth with a diagnosis then called gender identity disorder and seventeen cisgender boys. The average age of children in the study was eight. The researchers subsequently asked college students to rate the children on how "attractive," "handsome," and "beautiful" they were on scales from one to five. It was, disturbingly, a hot-or-not for children.

The researchers found that college students rated children with gender identity disorder as prettier than the cisgender boys. While some have interpreted this to mean that Stoller was right, the obvious alternative explanation is that the kids with so-called gender identity disorder altered their appearances (haircuts and so forth) to look more feminine to match their gender identity. Another possibility is that the same innate biological factors that made them identify as female also resulted in their facial features appearing more "feminine." Nothing in the study established that their social environments made them transgender.

A few years later, the same researchers conducted an identical study of children assigned female at birth with "gender identity disorder." They found that college students rated the children in the study with "gender identity disorder" as less beautiful than cisgender girls. Again, the study didn't prove that the environment made kids transgender, but it sent a message to transgender boys that they were unattractive, promoting an offensive theory with the potential to diminish the self-esteem of already marginalized children.

Zucker and Bradley also wondered if trauma was the cause of trans masculine identities. In one case, they theorized that a transgender boy "became transgender" because of his father's chronic anger, calling the boy's gender identity a kind of Stockholm syndrome in which he identified with the aggressor. They also wondered whether youths assigned female at birth who were sexually abused would identify as male to try to escape the possibility of being sexually assaulted again. In discussing a study in which researchers found no evidence that sexual trauma changed gender identity, Zucker and Bradley argued that the abuse "may not have been severe enough to impair the girls' core sense of themselves as female." In the end, no study has convincingly shown that being transgender is a result of trauma.*

---

* Some individuals may choose, within the confines of a safe and supportive psychotherapy environment, to explore the intricate relationships between trauma and the way they think about their gender. With the caveat that there is no convincing evidence that trauma causes trans identities, I will let people know that this is an idea they may encounter on social media or other media outlets and ask their reactions to the notion. I find it helpful for them to have encountered this notion in a supportive environment, prior to starting gender-affirming medical interventions, rather than after, given the stress and potential gaslighting it can cause if one were to hear this theory for the first time after starting a medical intervention.

Why did these researchers so doggedly pursue research into the possible environmental causes of being transgender? An underlying premise of their work is the idea that, if they could figure out what caused someone to be transgender, they could cure it—to put it simply, they presumed that being transgender was an illness to be fixed.

In all three instances we've looked at (autism, schizophrenia, and gender diversity), psychiatrists hinged their research on the belief that these conditions could and should be changed through talk therapy. Particularly when it came to gender diversity (and often with autism), this approach was flawed because it was labeling something that wasn't pathological as something that needed to be "fixed." But even if these psychiatrists were correct in thinking that it was reasonable to try to change someone's gender identity, and that identifying as transgender was the result of one's environment, this wouldn't necessarily make it reversible through talk therapy. Things being caused by the environment doesn't mean they are reversible through talk therapy. Many of these psychosocial theories around what makes someone transgender laid the groundwork for gender identity conversion efforts, in which therapists tried to force transgender people to be cisgender. The therapists thought moms being too close to their children made their kids transgender, so they recommended "letting go of [the child] by [the] mother." They thought that spending too much time with opposite-sex peers caused "gender identity disorder," so they recommended "decreasing play dates with [opposite-sex] peers." Those efforts didn't work, and research later showed that those subjected to them were more likely to attempt suicide.

PSEUDOSCIENCE TODAY:
THE NEW GENDER DIVERSITY BLAME GAME

People around Katie and her family were on a desperate search for what in the environment could have caused her to be transgender. They were hardly alone. In 2018, the blaming of social environments for gender diversity was revitalized under a new name: rapid-onset gender dysphoria. Dr. Lisa Littman, an obstetrician-gynecologist researcher at Brown University coined this term in a single-author publication in the scientific journal *PLoS One*. Sophisticated research studies usually involve a team of researchers, and a single-author research paper is unusual, particularly if the author in question has no prior expertise in the topic.

Dr. Littman reported the results of an anonymous survey of parents she recruited through three websites: 4thwavenow.com, transgendertrend.com, and youthtranscriticalprofessionals.org.*

Given where the survey respondents were recruited, the results of Dr. Littman's study were not surprising. These parents

---

* 4thwavenow is a reference to fourth-wave feminism, a feminist movement that emerged around 2012. Fourth-wave feminism has a small submovement of "trans-exclusionary radical feminists" who assert that transgender men are just women fleeing misogyny and that transgender women are men with nefarious goals trying to invade female spaces. The website describes itself as a gathering spot for parents who think their transgender children are not really transgender. Transgendertrend.com, as the name implies, is an organization of parents who similarly believe that transgender children are caught up in a "trend." The slogan on their website reads, "No child is born in the wrong body." The third website, youthtranscriticalprofessionals.org, is an organization whose members believe that transgender youth become transgender because of "binges on social media sites."

overwhelmingly believed that their children identified as trans-gender all of a sudden and that this identification coincided with their watching videos of transgender people online and linking up with new friends who were LGBTQ. Many of the parents also noted that their children suffered from mental health problems such as depression, and the study suggested that these adolescents' transgender identities were merely a result of their mental illness. (No logical explanation for why depression would make someone identify as transgender was provided.)

Based on these surveys, Dr. Littman proposed a new diag-nosis: rapid-onset gender dysphoria. She theorized that these children were cisgender, mentally ill, and confused. She sug-gested that they were influenced by social media and peer pres-sure that made them believe they were transgender, and that their trans identity was a maladaptive coping mechanism. She went so far as to compare their being transgender to dangerous behaviors some people use to cope, such as anorexia and cut-ting. It's worth noting that Dr. Littman had never taken care of transgender patients (a point she clarified when asked directly at the 2018 annual meeting of the American Academy of Child & Adolescent Psychiatry) and, being an obstetrician-gynecologist, is not a mental health professional.

As far as research methodology goes, the study was deeply flawed. All it showed was that parents on websites founded on the idea that social media makes kids transgender believed that social media made their kids transgender. In an interview with the *Economist*, Dr. Diane Ehrensaft, UCSF psychologist, professor of pediatrics, and a close colleague of mine, stated that Littman's methodology was akin to "recruiting from Klan or alt-right sites to demonstrate that people who are Black really are an inferior race."

The single most glaring issue with the study was that Dr. Littman did not interview any of the kids. What would they have had to say about their parents' claims regarding their gender identities?

When I sat down with Katie and told her about the study, she rolled her eyes: "That's the most bullshit thing ever." At that, her mom pushed her thick-rimmed glasses down on her nose and anxiously looked over at me. I assured her that Katie's swearing was okay—and certainly warranted. Katie explained that she could have easily looked like a kid with "rapid-onset gender dysphoria" to an outside observer but that none of Dr. Littman's presumptions would have applied.

To Katie's mom, it had seemed as if her daughter identified as transgender suddenly. Jillian remembers being shocked and thinking, "But you were never girlie. Where is this coming from?" From Jillian's perspective, it seemed as if Katie's identity had been "rapid onset."

Katie had known for many years before officially coming out that she didn't experience gender the way cisgender kids around her did, but since the tutu incident, she was terrified that people would discover her difference and that she would be harassed and rejected. In her elementary and middle schools, other kids would tease her when she slipped up and did something feminine. If she accidentally revealed that she liked pink, she'd be called a fairy. If she expressed too much natural emotion in drama class, boys would call her homophobic slurs. The hardest part of this for Katie was that she didn't understand what was going on with herself. She felt like a girl, but she had never heard the word *transgender*. Being a girl never seemed like an option, so she repressed her confusing feelings as much as she could.

When she entered high school, Katie had a eureka moment. On her first day of study hall, she walked into a crowded classroom. Kids everywhere were talking loudly, and she struggled to find a rickety desk that wasn't already taken. Through the chaos, she spotted a group of kids, one of whom was a boy sporting pink nail polish. She felt her heart race with excitement, and without thinking, she sat down with those students, who seemed to know one another from middle school (Katie had gone to a different one). They were friendly and introduced themselves to her. She learned that Julia, with her black pixie cut and angular features, was a cisgender lesbian. She liked to wear overalls with one strap hanging over her shoulder and was obsessed with cars. Daniel, who talked nonstop about the national tour of *Wicked* he had just seen, was gay and cisgender; he was the one with the hot-pink nails. Alex, who wore a Tennessee Titans jersey and looked like a typical football jock, was straight and cisgender and had two moms. The corners of Katie's mouth curled upward into a smile as she spoke with them. Who were these people?!

With this new group of friends, Katie finally stopped repressing her instincts. She spoke with a naturally higher voice. She admitted to them that she liked "girlie" things. At one point, Alex was talking to Julia about an episode of *I Am Jazz* he had watched the night before, a TLC show about a young transgender girl. Katie's ears perked up as she heard about Jazz. Up until that point, the only transgender people she had seen on TV usually played sex workers or murder victims on *Law &*

Order: SVU. For the first time, she was hearing about someone who was like her. Maybe it was possible to be an openly trans person.

Each day when she returned home, she would, in her words, "butch back up" and wouldn't let her parents know that she was expressing her feminine side at school. Her parents knew she had a new group of LGBTQ friends, but they assumed that Katie was just open-minded and friendly. She had always been a kind kid who wouldn't judge others.

At home, Katie continued to deepen her voice, avoided feminine activities, and never said a word about gender. So, when she ultimately opened up to her parents years later, it seemed as if it came out of nowhere. Katie remembers walking down to the family room where her parents were playing cards. She felt as if her throat were tied in a knot as she tried to say the words out loud. According to her mom, Katie's face lost all color and she looked horrified. She finally blurted out, "I think I'm transgender," and started to cry. Her parents were shocked and didn't at first know what to say. They told her that they would always love her and that they wanted some time to process.

In the words of Dr. Littman, Katie's news seemed "rapid onset" to her parents. Katie suspects this would have been even more dramatic for the kids in Littman's study: "If those kids knew their parents were prone to those kinds of beliefs, they'd be horrified to come out. When you spend years trying to hide something about yourself, you get pretty good at it. Of course their parents wouldn't have known before the kids wanted them to." Luckily, Katie's parents have been supportive. Though it took time for them to process and understand, they are now vocal and enthusiastic advocates for their child.

Our research team recently examined this question of how much time generally elapses between transgender people's coming to understand their gender identity and their telling another person. Analyzing a sample of over sixteen thousand transgender adults, we found that for people who first came to understand their gender identity in childhood, they didn't share this with another person for a median of fourteen years.

Over years of coming to understand herself, Katie also started watching videos about being transgender. Her friends played around with gender expression, but they were all cisgender. Daniel liked to paint his nails, but it was clear in his mind that he was a boy. Katie's new friends loved and accepted her, but they weren't quite experiencing the same thing as she was. Because there weren't any out transgender girls in her school, she looked online to better understand herself and find community. Social media had the added bonus of letting her be anonymous, so she didn't need to worry about being outed.* She watched YouTube videos of transgender people talking about their lives and transitioning. She learned a lot, but she emphasized to me that those videos didn't "make her" transgender. She sought them out because she wanted to learn

---

* As a member of the media committee of the American Academy of Child & Adolescent Psychiatry, I spend a lot of time thinking about the nuances of how media, and social media in particular, impact young people. For LGBTQ youth who don't have other LGBTQ youth around them, it can be an important lifeline for forming connection and belonging. However, not all online spaces are appropriately moderated and safe for minors. It's essential to teach youth about the dangers of talking to strangers online and to make sure their online spaces, and the way they are interacting online, are safe. The American Academy of Child & Adolescent Psychiatry has resources for parents to help them talk to their kids about their internet use.

more about herself and what being transgender meant. Her new group of friends also didn't make her transgender, but they provided a space where, for the first time, she felt safe being herself. She was, for the first time, being her authentic self and *belonging* instead of changing herself for the sake of *fitting in* to find connection.

As Katie explained to me, she also didn't become transgender because she was depressed. Rather, she attributes her many years of depression to being afraid that she wouldn't be accepted for being transgender. She added, "I can only imagine how much worse it would have been if my mom was on one of those websites." Kids and teens like Katie will be quick to tell you that social media didn't make them transgender, but their voices rarely make it into the national media the way those of political pundits do.

Dr. Littman's *PLoS One* survey received a surge of attention. *Wall Street Journal* columnist Abigail Shrier published an op-ed titled "When Your Daughter Defies Biology: The Burden of Mothers Whose Children Suffer from 'Rapid Onset Gender Dysphoria.'" In the op-ed, Shrier uncritically described Dr. Littman's theories as fact: kids were becoming transgender due to social media, and it was a mental illness. Shrier went on to write *Irreversible Damage: The Transgender Craze Seducing Our Daughters*, a book in which she interviewed parents like those from the websites Dr. Littman visited and left out their kids' voices. The *Economist* ran similar pieces warning people about rapid-onset gender dysphoria. A fringe idea became a full-fledged conspiracy theory. Every major medical organization said that being transgender wasn't a mental illness and that gender-affirming care should be made available to adolescents. The American

Psychological Association issued a statement outlining that rapid-onset gender dysphoria should not be used in clinical or diagnostic applications, given the lack of empirical support for its existence. But political pundits proposed that maybe all these independent medical organizations were just caught up in some sort of "transgender craze."

As conservative media continued to push this idea that social media were making kids transgender, the journal *PLoS One* received a barrage of complaints about the paper's poor methodology and the way it overstated the significance of its findings. The journal editors required Dr. Littman to revise the paper and issue a correction in which she explained that rapid-onset gender dysphoria was a theory rather than an established diagnosis. The correction also highlighted the fact that she had not interviewed any of the children themselves, nor their doctors, to get their views on whether social media and the environment made them transgender.

Soon after the 2018 paper was published, due to the scientific issues with the study, Brown University took down its press release about it. This resulted in a media frenzy around "academic censorship" that added fuel to the fire, giving the paper more and more attention. Ben Shapiro wrote a piece for the *Daily Wire* titled "A Brown University Researcher Released a Study about Teens Imitating Their Peers by Turning Trans. The Left Went Insane. So Brown Caved." Fox News ran headlines that Brown was "censoring" Littman. When Target and Amazon removed *Irreversible Damage* from their online stores, more media coverage followed, and Shrier found herself a regular on Fox News to talk about rapid-onset gender dysphoria. She was also invited to testify in front of Congress to oppose the

Equality Act, a federal bill that would outlaw discrimination against LGBTQ people.

Rapid-onset gender dysphoria was even cited in an amicus brief* for the Supreme Court case *Harris Funeral Homes v. Equal Opportunity Employment Commission*, which asked the Supreme Court whether Title VII's prohibition of discrimination based on sex in the realm of employment should be extended to transgender people. In one amicus brief, three sociologists essentially argued that many transgender people are suffering from rapid-onset gender dysphoria, and thus there is not a legal basis for extending federal employment protections to people who are transgender. One of these sociologists was Mark Regnerus, who is notorious for publishing a 2012 research study that claimed to find that children of gay parents are more likely to end up unemployed and dependent on social welfare programs (the paper was condemned by the American Sociological Association for weak methodology and spurious conclusions). His paper was funded by the conservative Witherspoon Institute and was used in the fight against marriage equality.

Eventually, media sources including *Scientific American* explained that rapid-onset gender dysphoria didn't have much basis in science. But the damage had been done. People around the world were convinced that transgender identity was caused by external social forces. And once again, the implication was that these identities were unacceptable, pathological, and should be "cured."

---

* This is sometimes called a "friend of the court" brief, in which interested parties weigh in on a court issue and submit their statements to the judges deciding the case.

Watching this all happen from California, I was relieved that my patients lived in a place where they were more accepted than in others. But they were still impacted by the media frenzy. Hearing powerful politicians say that their identities were just mental illness, even when they knew it wasn't true, impacted them. It worsened their self-esteem and in many instances their anxiety and depression. With all the rampant stigmatizing language spreading online and in the news, it seemed clear that social structures *supporting* trans kids weren't the problem— the problem was the historical, and now growing, social structures *attacking* trans kids. As one transgender teen in a focus group once told me, "If I am depressed or anxious, it's likely not because I have issues with my gender identity, but because everyone else does."

The good news amid the political chaos was that within medicine and the mental health profession, we were increasingly focusing on how to help these kids and their families. Almost universally, that meant providing emotional support and strategies to be resilient in the face of social and political attacks. For some of those families, it also meant considering gender-affirming medical interventions, which, though around for decades, were just starting to be more commonly available.

5

Puberty Blockers

Buying Time

The onset of puberty can be an important milestone for transgender youth. For some, they'll start the physical changes of their endogenous puberty* and be fine, other than the usual difficulties cisgender kids also face with puberty (acne, growth spurts, and so forth). But other transgender youth may develop severe psychological distress from their bodies developing in ways that don't align with their gender identity. This is the earliest stage at which medical professionals may consider any kind of gender-affirming medical care. That first

---

* As a reminder, *endogenous* means the puberty one would undergo without any external intervention.

step would be a puberty blocker—a medication that's been around since the 1980s and can temporarily put puberty on pause.

Three months after our first appointment, I noticed seven-year-old Sam had shown up on my clinic schedule again. Kate told the front desk that she wanted to have another check-in to make sure everything was going okay. I logged into Zoom, and there was Sam, cradling Squeakums in his arms. He giggled when the hamster tickled his arm with his whiskers, then sheepishly said hello. He still had long braids down to his shoulders, and his nails were purple today, the paint gently chipped around the edges.

I asked him how things had been since I saw him last, and he said pretty good. School was still fun, and he hadn't seen the bully Joey since the time Joey pushed him. In terms of gender, he still felt about the same—sometimes he felt more like a boy, sometimes he felt more like a girl, but this wasn't an issue from his perspective; he was just living his life however felt most authentic each day.

Sam's mom had told the front desk that she wanted me to look into how Sam was feeling about the prospect of going through his endogenous testosterone puberty sometime in the next few years. I asked Sam if he had ever heard the word *puberty* or learned about it in school or from his mom. He told me he had heard about it a little bit but didn't know very much. He said he would be okay talking about it and learning more, putting Squeakums down in his cage so he could listen more closely.

I told Sam that within the next few years his brain would start making chemicals that would tell his body to change in different ways, and that this is a normal healthy thing that happens for almost all kids. I pulled up the Zoom whiteboard and drew the outline of a generic person, then asked Sam to tell me what changes would happen to his body if he went through puberty today. He squinted one eye looking at the picture, then yelled, "My voice will change!," trying his best to simulate a deeper masculine voice. I drew a small music note next to the figure's face to denote the deepening of the voice that comes as testosterone thickens and lengthens the vocal cords.

I asked him if anything else would happen in the head part of the figure if he went through puberty, and Sam gave me a puzzled look. I told him that facial hair would eventually start to grow and pointed to my own stubble, then colored in a beard on the picture.

As we continued to fill out the picture together, we talked about all the changes from puberty: Adam's apple development, muscle growth, getting taller, acne, the whole thing. I carefully watched Sam's reactions as we talked about the puberty he would go through without any medical intervention. For some trans kids, they become sullen and scared when thinking about how their bodies will change. But Sam seemed to be taking in the information without much anxiety.

I then erased the board and drew another figure—this time asking Sam to tell me what a "girl puberty" would look like. He was able to tell me that there wouldn't be the same facial hair or Adam's apple growth and that there would be chest growth, which he drew on the figure himself. We talked about how the voice doesn't change in the same way for "girl puberty."

Throughout our whiteboard exercise, I realized that Sam knew more than he had initially let on. Though he didn't know the word *testosterone*, he knew what would come along with his own endogenous testosterone puberty (this sometimes comes as news to other young children I work with). When asked how he felt about that, he said he wasn't sure yet. I told him that was okay and to keep me and his mom updated if he had any new thoughts about it. We spent a few more minutes playing an unrelated *Pictionary* game to wind down, and he had me guess the word *snowman*, reminding me that he'd never seen one since he lived in a warmer part of California.

Once we finished the game, Sam brought the computer back to his mom. I let her know that Sam seemed to have a pretty good understanding of puberty and understood that without any intervention, he would go through a testosterone-driven puberty. He also didn't seem particularly stressed about the idea, which could indicate that he won't end up wanting or needing any medical interventions.

This is such an important point for parents to understand. There is no one way to be transgender, just as there's no one way to be cisgender. Some transgender people want medical interventions, and some don't. Some are distressed by puberty, some aren't. The existence of one type of person doesn't invalidate the existence of the other. It was also entirely possible that Sam's understanding of his gender would continue to evolve, and he might ultimately feel that the *cisgender* label fits best for him, or potentially a *nonbinary* label.

I did let Kate know, however, that it could also be that he's still processing the information or that things could change once he started puberty. For now, all we needed to do was watch and see how things evolved. I let Kate know that she was far ahead of the vast majority of parents in making sure she was doing everything she could to make sure Sam was supported. For most kids, these conversations around gender and puberty never happen.

As I closed the Zoom call, I couldn't help but think about how Sam and Kate brought the research of Dr. Caitlin Ryan, from San Francisco State University, to life. Dr. Ryan is a social worker and director of the Family Acceptance Project, a research and intervention program that helps families support the mental health of racially, ethnically, and religiously diverse LGBTQ children. In one seminal study by Dr. Ryan's research team, published in the *Journal of Child and Adolescent Psychiatric Nursing* in 2010, her team surveyed 245 LGBTQ young adults and measured their mental health, as well as the degree to which their families had supported their LGBTQ identities. Measures of family support included such questions as "How often did any of your parents/caregivers appreciate your clothing or hairstyle, even though it might not have been typical for your gender?" Dr. Ryan's research team found that young adults with high levels of family acceptance of their LGBTQ identities and diverse gender expressions were nearly half as likely to have attempted suicide. They also had dramatically better scores on measures of depression, substance use, self-esteem, and overall health.

One major point that came away from Dr. Ryan's work was that parents almost universally want what is best for their kid. However, many think that trying to push their children to fit in and conform to society's gendered expectations is what will help them thrive, because they will be "fitting in." But Dr. Ryan's research, through clear data, shows this just isn't the case. That forced fitting in just leads to shame and a whole host of bad downstream effects (anxiety, depression, substance use, and even considering suicide). On the other hand, she found that expressing love when your child comes out, advocating for your child when the child is bullied or picked on for being gender diverse, and standing up to family members who are critical of your child's gender expression, all help young people to grow up to be mentally healthy, confident, and strong.

Sadly, this kind of open acceptance of a child's gender expression isn't common. It has been documented internationally that young people are shamed and harassed when acting like themselves doesn't line up with societal expectations based on their sex assigned at birth. In October of 2017, the *Journal of Adolescent Health* published a special issue on how sex and gender influence young people around the world. In the issue, a team of researchers reported on their analysis of in-depth interviews of 129 adolescents in two "middle-income cities" (Shanghai, China, and New Delhi, India) and two "high-income cities" (Baltimore, United States, and Ghent, Belgium). They found that across all four cultures, children who challenged gender norms were bullied. They were laughed at, gossiped about, and called names. The bullying was more common against those assigned male at birth (like Sam) than those assigned female at birth, though both groups were intensely harassed.

Noting that rejection of gender diversity is a cross-cultural problem, Dr. Ryan's group has also begun creating materials that are culturally tailored to help families understand and support their gender diverse children—focusing on which "accepting behaviors" her research has tied to better mental health outcomes and which "rejecting behaviors" her research has tied to worse mental health outcomes.* These include materials in English, Spanish, and Mandarin. She's also created materials tailored toward specific religious groups, including the Church of Jesus Christ of Latter-day Saints.

Family support is vital and protective. For some kids it is all they need. But some other transgender kids struggle with severe psychological reactions to the ways in which their bodies develop during puberty.

As a medical student, I would get on an Amtrak train every month between New Haven and Boston so that I could visit the first medical clinic in the United States for transgender youth: the Gender Multispecialty Service (GeMS) at Boston Children's Hospital, the pediatric teaching hospital of Harvard Medical School. I have fond memories of sitting on the old trains and watching snow fall over the New England landscape while I cozied up and read research papers about the medical interventions GeMS was using—puberty blockers and gender-affirming hormones like estrogen and testosterone for adolescents struggling with gender dysphoria.

Boston Children's Hospital is a true behemoth, with over four hundred pediatric hospital beds and world experts in just about every area of pediatric medicine. It has been ranked as

---

* For those who are interested, materials from the Family Acceptance Project are available at https://familyproject.sfsu.edu/.

the best pediatric medical center in the United States by *U.S. News & World Report* more times than any other hospital in the country.

I remember walking into the lobby the first day in my khakis, dress shirt, and medical-school-issued short white coat, trying to find my way to the gender clinic. As I walked up the stairs, I noticed each one singing, a different note chiming every time my loafer landed on a new step.

It was in that hospital that I met Dr. Norman Spack, the pediatric endocrinologist who founded the GeMS clinic formally in 2007 (though he had been treating trans patients with gender-affirming medical care going back to at least 1998). By the time I met Dr. Spack, he was an associate professor of pediatrics and a widely respected pediatric endocrinologist. He wore a traditional long white coat with a collared shirt and tie underneath and maintained a neatly trimmed goatee that surrounded his gregarious smile. He spoke with an accent that combined his Massachusetts roots with the academic diction that comes from working in the Harvard system for decades.

The first time I visited Dr. Spack in his clinic, he brought me with him to meet one of his new patients, a sixteen-year-old transgender girl named Cara. When we walked into the exam room, I saw Cara sitting on a medical exam table wearing a blue checkered gown, her light gray eyes unfocused. Her forearms were covered in faint healed scars from where she had cut herself when feeling overwhelmed. Like many other kids who struggle with overwhelmingly intense feelings of anxiety and depression, Cara had turned to the cutting in an attempt to make some of those overwhelming feelings go away when nothing else would work.* Later, by engaging with therapy, she was finally able to stop by replacing that behavior with other stress-relief techniques like deep breathing and tensing and relaxing her muscles.

Dr. Spack began by talking to Cara about how her weekend was and what she was planning to do over the upcoming summer break, before diving into what kind of help she was seeking around gender. Cara shared with us that she felt so dysphoric about her genitals developing that she willed herself not to go to the bathroom for extended periods of time. She was afraid of going to the bathroom because she would have to wipe, and that would mean looking at her penis. She didn't go to the bathroom for so long that her intestines perforated, which required surgery. Luckily, she had recovered okay, but she realized that she couldn't keep going on the way she was going, without any kind of gender-affirming medical care. She had read about medications that could have stalled her puberty and prevented this distress, but she suspected it was too late for one, since she had progressed so far through puberty. She had been seeing a therapist who specializes in gender over the past year and had a letter from that therapist explaining that estrogen would likely help her distress. She wanted to talk about what taking that medication would mean and when she could start.

---

* Of note, nonsuicidal self-injury such as cutting serves different functions for different people. Some of my patients tell me it serves a self-punishing purpose, some tell me it alleviates difficult emotions, and others tell me it makes them feel something when they are feeling numb. It can be an extraordinarily difficult behavior to stop and a dangerous one. The most effective treatment for this is a therapy called dialectical behavioral therapy.

Cara's situation reminded me a lot of Kyle, who I had met in the emergency room. He'd told me that as his puberty progressed, he became miserable. His chest was a constant painful reminder of his body not lining up with the boy he knew he was, and he started restricting his eating to try to flatten his chest and stop his periods. Showering was nearly impossible, and he avoided it anytime he could. He layered on multiple sports bras and used tape to try to flatten his chest, up until the point he could barely breathe. While some companies sell safe clothing for trans masculine and non-binary people that's designed to give their chest a flatter contour, Kyle didn't have access to this. In a 2016 study of eighteen hundred trans people who bound their chest, 97 percent had at least one health-related problem from binding. Common issues included back pain (54 percent), over-heating (54 percent), chest pain (49 percent), and shortness of breath (47 percent); 2.8 percent told the researchers that binding resulted in a rib fracture. These kinds of problems could have been avoided had these young people had earlier access to puberty blockers, which would have paused chest development, giving them more time to explore their gender identities and next steps. These issues with chest binding can also be avoided if a person follows certain guidelines. We usually recommend that patients purchase their binder from a trusted company (gc2b is one of the most popular), make sure the binder isn't too tight (one should be able to fit two fingers between the binder and the skin), never wear a binder for more than eight consecutive hours, and don't sleep in a binder. Children's Hospital Los Angeles has put together a useful resource with more information on safe binding practices.*

While some political pundits have voiced opposition to gender-affirming top surgery (surgery to remove chest tissue and create a flatter contour for trans masculine and nonbinary adolescents), they also generally oppose puberty blockers, despite the fact that puberty blockers could prevent the need for future chest surgeries if offered at the appropriate time. Notably, though politicians in many U.S. states have tried to ban gender-affirming medical care for transgender adolescents, particularly chest surgery, they have not attempted to outlaw breast surgeries for cisgender minors, despite these surgeries for cisgender minors being relatively common. For example, the American Society of Plastic Surgeons highlighted that almost six thousand teenage cisgender girls and three thousand teenage cisgender boys had aesthetic breast reductions in 2022.

When we left the exam room, Dr. Spack let out a deep sigh. Cara was right, a puberty blocker would have prevented many of the physical changes she'd experienced with puberty. But based on Dr. Spack's physical exam, most of her puberty was already finished. Though the blocker would obviously not have gotten rid of her penis that was causing distress, it would have decreased the frequency of spontaneous erections, which bothered Cara, as well as many of the other physical changes that would now be difficult if not impossible to

---

* This resource is available at https://www.chla.org/sites/default/files/atoms/files/ Binding_English%20parent.pdf.

reverse: deepening of her voice, changes in bone structure, and the other list of testosterone-driven physical features Cara had shared with us that were bothering her. Dr. Spack reviewed the letter from Cara's therapist and asked a few other members of the team to join her in the room to talk more in depth about starting estrogen.

The clinic schedules at GeMS tended to be packed, and Dr. Spack brought me straight to the adjacent exam room to see his next patient. He introduced me to Veronica, a trans woman now in her early twenties who had received a puberty-blocking medication from the very beginning of her puberty. She had been on estrogen for years now and told Dr. Spack everything was going well. She told us that she had just landed a new job at a law office. She then turned to the man standing next to her and said, "We also got engaged!"

Dr. Spack lit up, "Oh my goodness, mazel tov!"

I remember sitting quietly in the clinic's conference room after these back-to-back appointments. The contrast could not have been more dramatic. This was in the mid-2010s, and Veronica really challenged the predominant narrative about transgender people at the time—the media constantly portrayed trans people as suffering, depressed, impoverished. But with medical and social support, Veronica was thriving.

Dr. Spack came into the conference room a few minutes later and handed me a small pile of papers that I realized was an article from the journal *European Child & Adolescent Psychiatry* called "Pubertal Delay as an Aid in Diagnosis and Treatment of a Transsexual Adolescent."

The paper had been published in 1998 and told the story of a patient named B who was around age nineteen at the time the paper was published. The authors of the paper explained that B, who was assigned a female sex at birth, had expressed identifying as a boy since he was a child. When he was twelve, his mother found a suicide note saying that B did not want to continue to live if he would need to enter his endogenous puberty. His parents took him to a local mental health clinic for talk therapy. This improved his depression somewhat, but he continued to be distraught at the prospect of puberty, afraid of his body betraying who he was. At age thirteen, his psychiatrist and a pediatric endocrinologist treated B with triptorelin. This medication binds to the part of the brain that is responsible for initiating puberty, turning it off. The authors of the paper noted that such puberty blockers were particularly appealing because they are reversible. If B were to change his mind and want to undergo his endogenous puberty, the medication could be stopped.

Triptorelin belongs to a class of medications called gonadotropin-releasing hormone analogs, or GnRH analogs for short. They are often colloquially called puberty blockers, blockers, or pubertal suppression. Puberty begins when a brain region called the hypothalamus starts to release spurts of a hormone called GnRH. It releases the hormone in periodic bursts, and this pulsatile release tells another part of the brain—the anterior pituitary—to make hormones called luteinizing hormone (LH) and follicle-stimulating hormone (FSH). Those hormones then tell either the testes or ovaries to make testosterone or estrogen respectively. With this, puberty begins.

GnRH analogs look chemically similar to the GnRH made by the hypothalamus. They make the anterior pituitary think that GnRH levels are constantly high.* Because the pulsatile release of GnRH is no longer perceived by the pituitary, it stops making FSH and LH, shutting down the whole cascade needed for puberty to progress. If the GnRH analog is stopped, the pulsatile release from the hypothalamus returns, and puberty proceeds again as if the medication had never been there.

These medications have been around for decades and used in many areas of medicine. Because prostate cancer grows when exposed to testosterone, they can be used for older people with prostate cancer to slow its progression. They have also been used for children who enter puberty very early due to a condition called central precocious puberty. Some of these young people enter puberty as young as ages two or three. A series of papers in the 1980s showed that these medications could effectively and temporarily pause puberty for such young people.

The authors of the paper Dr. Spack had handed me explained that B felt some relief after starting the triptorelin, which allowed him to engage more with his therapist, without the pressure of any physical developments from puberty, which B was aware would require surgery to undo, if they could be undone at all.

Though the paper is somewhat vague as to the nature of B's talk therapy, it notes that once B realized his gender identity

---

* This fine scientific point can be confusing. Many people think that puberty blockers are GnRH antagonists (meaning they block the receptor), but they are actually GnRH agonists (meaning they activate the receptor). The reason they work is that the receptor needs to sense pulsatile activation for the pituitary to make FSH and LH, and constant activation prevents it from proceeding with the downstream effects of puberty.

would not become female, he stopped going. He continued to suffer with a great deal of shame around being "transsexual" (the term used at the time), and his parents also were uncomfortable with the idea of his trans identity.

Eventually, the family reached out to a specialized clinic for trans people in the Netherlands, what is now called the VUMC Center of Expertise on Gender Dysphoria. This is where the family met the authors of the paper. The psychologists from their group continued to help B deal with the feelings of shame around being trans and to work on his self-esteem. They supported B and his parents with family therapy, particularly focused on his dad's difficulty coming to terms with B's being transgender. And B participated in some groups with other young trans masculine people, helping him to see that trans people "can be just like other peers," as the paper put it.

At age eighteen,* B started taking testosterone to induce male puberty. The authors of the paper noted that B became more "easy going and friendly" after testosterone. Once he had reached the age of majority in the Netherlands, he underwent masculinizing chest surgery to create a more male chest contour, as well as surgery to remove his ovaries and uterus.

When the doctors from the clinic followed up with B a year after the surgeries, B reported that he felt great. He had no regrets about his medical decisions, was happy with his life, and was studying to become a physician himself.

The story of B seemed to mirror that of Veronica. And

---

* The paper notes that B chose this timing so that he could start testosterone after high school was finished and he was moving into a new phase of his life.

both stories were in stark contrast to what Cara had gone through.

After the Dutch group published their paper, more and more physicians began adopting their approach of providing puberty blockers to transgender adolescents. Dr. Spack himself sent members of his team to Amsterdam to learn about the Dutch group's protocol, which he later brought to Boston Children's Hospital, where he created the GeMS program. Physicians from around the country looking to establish pediatric gender clinics in the United States subsequently traveled to Boston to train with Dr. Spack.

One thing that the doctors at VUMC emphasized was that they conducted a psychological assessment prior to initiating pubertal suppression. In their clinic, they had a team of mental health professionals who could meet with young people and their families to better understand their gender identities and desire to start pubertal suppression. The professionals would also ensure that the parents and the adolescents understood exactly what these medications do and don't do, as well as all the side effects patients could encounter. The team would speak to the families and the adolescents at length, helping them think through what it would be like for the youths to change their gender expression: How would people around them react? How would they feel? Was there anything they were worried about that should be focused on before starting?

When Dr. Spack was setting up his clinic in the United States, he didn't have the same resources as the Dutch clinic—he couldn't hire a large team of mental health professionals to spend extended time with each patient prior to initiating a pubertal suppression. To deal with this problem, the clinic required that families come to them with what is now commonly referred to as "the letter." The letter would be written by a licensed mental health professional outside of the clinic who had worked with the patient at length. It would document that the patient met criteria for the gender-related diagnosis from the American Psychiatric Association's *Diagnostic and Statistical Manual of Mental Disorders* (the diagnosis was gender identity disorder in older editions; the new edition has the related diagnosis called gender dysphoria). The therapists would also document that they thought it was in the best interest of the adolescent to start pubertal suppression. Once families arrived at GeMS with a letter, GeMS had its own small team of psychologists who would work with the family to complete an additional long battery of assessments prior to initiating treatment. Most in the field are now skeptical of this extra battery of assessments, as it's unclear that all the hours of psychometrics by an additional psychologist are necessary, and this may carry the risk of further creating barriers to care and making young people feel stigmatized.

Since the so-called Dutch model was first described, the letter requirement itself has also garnered some controversy in the field. At the time of my writing, all major clinical guidelines require that trans youth have a psychological evaluation (the basis of the letter) prior to starting a puberty blocker. But some experts have pointed out that this requirement creates issues. As the Dutch noted in their case of B, the main reason to start B's blocker was to prevent the irreversible changes of puberty, while "extending the diagnostic period." That is, the medication wasn't meant to be a final treatment for their gender dysphoria, but rather a way to buy them more time to figure things out without the stress of puberty progressing. The Dutch seemed to have realized that while the puberty blocker was reversible, puberty itself was not. As we saw with Cara, the negative impact of an irreversible puberty could potentially be devastating.

When the GeMS clinic first established their letter requirement, adolescents and their families needed to have worked with the therapist for six months prior to the therapist writing the letter. You can imagine that this created problems for the kids who were actively progressing through puberty and watching their bodies change in ways that would be difficult to undo later.

The six-month requirement was relatively arbitrary—it was a number that came from the *Diagnostic and Statistical Manual of Mental Disorders* itself—an estimate of how long doctors would want to see an adolescent identify as transgender before feeling comfortable that such an identity was probably stable and unlikely to change in the future.

Because clinical guidelines, set forth by the Endocrine Society and the World Professional Association for Transgender Health (WPATH), require such a psychological evaluation, clinics around the world continue to require it, but the process of creating the letter varies somewhat by clinic. Though the content of the letter tends to be more or less the same, different therapists have different ideas regarding how long a patient needs to be in care with them before they will write it. While patients would need to have identified as a gender different from their sex assigned at birth for at least six months to meet gender dysphoria diagnostic criteria, some therapists will take a history from the parents and the adolescent to establish that this has been true for the past six months, rather than the therapists themselves needing to witness this for six months.

Another reason for the push to shorten this diagnostic period prior to starting a puberty blocker was that wait lists for gender therapists and gender clinics have been extraordinarily long. A patient could feasibly wait several months to find a gender therapist with an opening, undergo six months of therapy to get a letter, then wait another year or longer to actually get in to see a physician who would prescribe the puberty blocker. By that point, many patients may have already completed puberty, and the puberty blocker would have lost most of its utility.

During the early years of the GeMS clinic seeing patients, a second clinic for trans youth opened in Rhode Island, led by the Brown School of Medicine assistant dean of admissions and adolescent medicine physician Dr. Michelle Forcier.

The first time I sat down with Dr. Forcier, we were both speaking at an annual meeting of the American Academy of Child & Adolescent Psychiatry. I immediately noticed a different presence from Dr. Spack's. Dr. Forcier had a big warm smile, a casual demeanor, and a bright blue highlight in her short curly hair. The day of her presentation, she wore a flowing bohemian dress. She's not one to use medical jargon, and her presentation was exceptionally clear.

When I spoke with her again years later, she shared with me that this casual demeanor, blue hair, and the fact that she's a woman mean that she's been brushed off by some of her colleagues in the past, despite her academic pedigree and status as a medical school assistant dean of admissions. They rarely ask her why she has the blue hair—the answer being that she knows it makes her less scary and more relatable to the kids for whom she cares.

It was clear when I spoke to her that she had a deep knowledge of the field of gender, but that her perspective was also unique. From her vantage point, many of the early gender clinics had implemented strict "assessment protocols" not because they were worried about their patients, but because they were worried about themselves. They wanted to be sure that 100 percent of the patients they saw would continue on the path of gender-affirming hormones. From her perspective, it seemed they were driven by a fear that if a single patient didn't continue to identify as trans in the future, there would be a negative media storm, or a malpractice case, and that it would hurt the physicians.

"But what about the patients?" she asked me. She would see a large number of patients who were turned away from the GeMS clinic because their cases were complex: adolescents who also had autism, adolescents with a history of trauma, adolescents whose families couldn't afford a prolonged course of therapy or whose children were so distressed by puberty that they feared their mental health would deteriorate dramatically if they had to wait through six months of active therapy before even being able to get in line to wait for a puberty blocker.

Dr. Forcier still conducted a mental health assessment for all patients starting gender-affirming medical interventions, including puberty blockers. Trained in adolescent medicine, she was able to sit with a family herself and create what's called a biopsychosocial formulation, in which she considered all the biological factors, psychological factors, and social factors relevant to a family. In some cases, she would talk to the family and decide that the case was too complex from a mental health perspective. In those cases, she would inform the family that it was in their best interests to continue with therapy prior to any medical intervention. But in other cases, it would be clear from her conversations with the family and the adolescent that, weighing the risks and benefits, starting pubertal suppression without waiting for six months of therapy was the best way to go.

At the end of the day, we don't have a clear data-driven answer regarding the utility of requiring a biopsychosocial assessment and mental health letter prior to starting pubertal suppression. For just about every other medical intervention in pediatrics, we don't take this approach. Instead, we take an "informed consent" approach, in which the parents and adolescent are told, by the prescribing doctor, all the risks, benefits, and potential side effects of the medication. The family then weighs these and decides on the best course of action for their adolescent child. Usually, an additional mental health professional doesn't need to be involved.

While letters are primarily designed to reduce regret rates, the fact that pubertal suppression itself is reversible makes this seem like a less important factor here when compared to the use of, say, estrogen and testosterone, which have more clear and often permanent physical effects. And the delay that letters can cause often means that kids miss the window for a puberty blocker that can offer immense relief. While these debates continue, it's worth highlighting that we may have a more data-driven answer soon. An NIH-funded four-site study of the impact of gender-affirming medical care includes one clinic with a more intensive assessment protocol, as well as one that follows more of an informed-consent model (with the adolescent-medicine doctor or pediatric endocrinologist conducting the biopsychosocial assessment rather than an additional mental health professional). Both clinics are following patients over time, and the study may reveal if one approach results in better outcomes than the other.

Despite these challenges and controversies regarding the degree of psychological assessment needed prior to starting puberty blockers, pediatric gender clinics in addition to GeMS popped up around the country, and doctors continued to study the mental health impacts of these interventions. Most of these clinics were at academic medical centers, where doctors tracked the mental health of adolescents who received gender-affirming medical care.

As I write this, there are at least eight research studies examining the impact of pubertal suppression on the mental health of transgender youth. Most have linked this intervention to better mental health outcomes. These studies include some from the original Dutch clinic, which linked access to puberty blockers to lower rates of depression and anxiety; a study from the United Kingdom that found improvements in overall mental health functioning; and a study from our group when I was at Harvard Medical School that found that those who accessed puberty blockers during adolescence had lower odds of considering suicide in their life when compared to those who desired blockers but weren't able to access them.

Some critics of gender-affirming medical care have noted that there have not been any double-blind, randomized, placebo-controlled trials of puberty blockers. Such a clinical trial is often considered the gold standard for evidence of an intervention being efficacious. This kind of study would require randomly giving adolescents with gender dysphoria either a puberty blocker or a placebo. However, most doctors feel that because of the level of evidence that we have, giving young people with clinically significant gender dysphoria a placebo would be unethical. For that reason, it doesn't seem that any university ethics board would approve such a study. Additionally, because puberty blockers have obvious physical impacts, "blinding" participants and researchers from whether a young person received the medication or a placebo would be impossible.

Some have asked whether studies have shown that kids who get blockers merely have better health because they have families that are more loving and supportive, raising the question of whether the mental health improvements were from the medications themselves. However, studies from our group and others have statistically controlled for level of family support, isolating the improvement in mental health to the puberty blockers themselves.

Others have asked whether, because so many of these kids receiving pubertal suppression are in talk therapy, if it's actually the talk therapy improving their mental health, rather than the puberty blockers. One of the best studies to look at this question was by Rosalia Costa and colleagues, published in the *Journal of Sexual Medicine* in 2015. This study followed two groups of kids: one group that was determined immediately eligible for puberty blockers, and a second group that was determined to not yet be eligible (some needed more time to make the decision as they worked through other mental health difficulties). Both groups received supportive psychotherapy alone for the first six months, and for the not-yet-eligible group, their mental health improved.* From this we can seem to conclude that supportive therapy (supporting kids through conflict with peers around gender, helping the family validate and accept their child, and so forth) can be helpful for general mental health. For the next year, the immediately eligible group received pubertal suppression and ongoing therapy, while the other group continued to receive therapy only. The group that continued to receive therapy only had their mental health plateau, with no further improvements. The group that received puberty blockers with therapy, however, saw their mental health steadily improve, suggesting that though therapy alone can be helpful for co-occurring mental health challenges other than gender dysphoria, puberty blockers are needed to truly improve mental health when adolescents are suffering from physical gender dysphoria. Most experts in the field will agree that this is what they experience in their day-to-day work with transgender youth suffering from physical gender dysphoria.†

That being said, every medical intervention is individualized and must cater to the unique patient in front of the

---

* The "immediately eligible" group, which was impacted by gender dysphoria but didn't appear to have other mental health challenges, didn't have mental health improvement over this period, suggesting that the supportive talk therapy wasn't helpful for gender dysphoria itself.

† Two other studies, one by Tordoff et al. in the journal *JAMA Network Open* and another by Achielle et al. in the *International Journal of Pediatric Endocrinology*, similarly found that mental health improvements from gender-affirming medical interventions could be separated out from the beneficial effects of psychotherapy.

doctor. Physicians, adolescents, and their families work with their doctors on a case-by-case basis to determine what the best medical option is for a given family.

Meredith, the teen from New England, and her mom, Suzanne, the professor, spent years contemplating pubertal suppression. For Meredith, who had been talking to her therapist and endocrinologist about the decision for two years, the choice to start the medication was clear.

Most of the conversations Meredith, Dr. Carey (her therapist), and her family had around puberty blockers were straightforward. Because one needs the sex hormones of puberty to mineralize and strengthen the bones, Meredith knew she would fall behind on bone density while on the medication. Dr. Stenton (her endocrinologist) would monitor her bones closely with dual-energy X-ray absorptiometry (DEXA) scans to make sure she would be safe from fractures. Research was somewhat mixed regarding whether Meredith would regain normal bone density after either stopping the blocker or starting estrogen, but the gap in bone mineral density wasn't substantial enough to suggest she would be at a high risk of a fracture. However, if she were to stay on the blocker indefinitely, this fracture risk would continue to increase, so Dr. Stenton recommended that they plan to make a decision to either stop the blocker or start estrogen by around age sixteen. Dr. Stenton also recommended that Meredith take vitamin D and calcium supplements and continue exercising, all of which promote healthy bone development.

Though it wasn't relevant to Meredith, it's worth noting that the Endocrine Society guidelines also briefly mention a phenomenon in which people assigned female at birth can experience menopause-like symptoms when they start puberty blockers. Over the years, physicians have noticed that when people assigned female at birth received puberty blockers later rather than earlier in their puberty, the drop in estrogen can cause hot flashes.

Dr. Stenton also reviewed with Meredith and Suzanne the Endocrine Society's comment that the impact of puberty blockers on brain development has only been preliminarily studied. There had been one study of the impact of puberty blockers on executive functioning (the set of cognitive skills important for planning and breaking down complex tasks) that found puberty blockers were not harmful to this aspect of cognition, but researchers had not yet studied every cognitive domain.

I personally have always found the text about cognitive functioning side effects in the guidelines a bit unusual, since we don't have this kind of data for the vast majority of medications we use in pediatrics. It has been my experience that puberty blockers, because they have been so hotly politicized, are held to a different standard than other medications. The informed consent or assessment process that we go through for puberty blockers is much more in depth than that for any other medication we prescribe, despite blockers being one of the more benign interventions used in pediatric medicine. Clinicians rarely go into the same level of depth and assessment with families when using the medication for its other indication—central precocious puberty (the condition in which youth enter puberty at an unusually young age).

The reality is that there are risks, benefits, and unknowns for all medications. We just tend to focus on the risks and unknowns much more for medications that are emotionally charged and heavily politicized. At the end of the day, medicine always involves weighing all these factors for a given individual and doing our best as physicians and parents to choose which intervention is *most likely* to result in the best outcome, based on what we know. In clinical medicine, we never know for sure what an outcome will be for a given patient. Medicine is a field of probabilities, not certainties.

I sometimes give the example of the medication Lipitor (atorvastatin), which is used for high cholesterol. Research shows that this medication reduces the risk of a heart attack or stroke. But it can also cause a rare side effect called rhabdomyolysis, in which your muscles break down, and the little bits of muscle clog and damage the kidneys.

We also haven't measured how Lipitor impacts every single cognitive domain. Yet as in all of medicine, we weigh the risks, benefits, and unknowns and choose what is most likely to help the patient. For those with very high cholesterol, taking the medication usually makes the most sense.

While most of the conversations around the risks and benefits of puberty blockers for Meredith and her family seemed straightforward, one topic was more complicated: fertility. Based on decades of experience using puberty blockers for precocious puberty, physicians are confident that they do not have a substantial impact on fertility. However, there is a strong theoretical risk that going straight from pubertal suppression to gender-affirming hormones (estrogen or testosterone) will result in infertility. Though it hasn't been studied in sufficient detail, clinical guidelines work on the assumption that this is the case. For that reason, and because most adolescents choose to go straight from puberty blockers to hormones, guidelines recommend fertility counseling and, for interested families, freezing eggs or sperm prior to starting a puberty blocker.

Meredith had explained to me during our first meeting the many reasons she didn't think banking sperm made sense, but Suzanne was worried. What if Meredith changed her mind in the future? Would she blame Suzanne for letting her forgo banking sperm?

Meredith's undergoing fertility preservation would be no small matter. She would need to interact with her genitals, which caused her severe emotional distress. She was also put off by the cost, which wasn't covered by insurance. Her family would need to pay about $1,000 up front, then $300 every year for the duration of the freezing. While her family could afford it, it seemed like an unnecessary cost to her.

Often, the decision to undergo fertility preservation is even harder for those assigned female at birth. The process for them requires a series of hormone injections, ultrasounds to track progress (usually through the vagina, though some newer techniques may be able to avoid this), and removal of the eggs, while under sedation. A single cycle of this can cost up to $10,000, with another $1,000 per year in storage fees. Sometimes, multiple cycles are needed before doctors are able to collect enough eggs.

Suzanne found herself troubled by some of the research about trans youth and fertility preservation. Meredith's perspective of not wanting to bank sperm seemed common among trans kids. In a 2017 study in the *Journal of Adolescent Health* of seventy-two transgender adolescents who underwent fertility counseling prior to starting gender-affirming medical care, only two (2.8 percent) opted for fertility preservation. Both were trans girls. Another study published in 2020 in the journal *JAMA Pediatrics* examined the medical records of one hundred and two adolescents and found that none of the forty-nine adolescents assigned female at birth chose to undergo fertility preservation, though more of the adolescents assigned male at birth like Meredith did: thirty-three of fifty-three (62 percent).

Suzanne worried about this because some studies of transgender adults showed higher rates of desiring biological children—roughly half. Other studies of transgender youth also showed much higher rates of wanting biological children— as high as 36 percent—which seemed in contrast to the low numbers of those who actually underwent fertility preservation. Was Meredith just feeling guilty about the cost?

Both Meredith and her mother realized that it was impossible to know with absolute certainty how Meredith would feel in the future about wanting children who were genetically related to her, but her reasoning for not wanting to undergo fertility preservation also made a lot of sense to Suzanne: not wanting to deal with the dysphoria of providing a sample, finding it somewhat unlikely that she would be in a relationship with someone who could provide an egg (though possible if she ended up with a trans man or nonbinary person), and feeling a strong connection to the idea of adoption. They decided that it was okay to push off the decision for now and to address it again prior to starting estrogen. If at that point Meredith felt strongly about wanting to undergo fertility preservation, she could stop the blocker, progress somewhat through her endogenous puberty, and bank sperm prior to starting the estrogen, which would likely impact her fertility.*

After all these discussions, Meredith finally had the appointment to have her puberty blocker placed. Dr. Stenton ordered a medication similar to triptorelin called histrelin.

One of the most commonly used versions of histrelin is a small rod implant that goes just under the skin of the arm.† It looks similar to Nexplanon birth control implants that many people use. Unless the rod is removed, it is marketed by the company to work for a year before a new one is needed, though some research has shown that it tends to last closer to two years.

Meredith and Suzanne arrived at the doctor's office for their 8:00 a.m. appointment and sat eagerly in the waiting room. Right at eight, a nurse brought them back to the procedure room and took Meredith's blood pressure and heart rate.

Dr. Stenton came in and asked Meredith if she was ready. She said yes and lay back on the exam table with her arm stretched out to the side. Dr. Stenton told her she would feel a small pinch as the doctor injected lidocaine to numb the area. Dr. Stenton then took out the histrelin implant placement device, which looked like a stapler with a long needle coming out of it. She pushed the needle into the plane

---

* It's worth noting here again that the clinical guidelines recommending fertility preservation are based on a strong suspicion mechanistically that going straight from pubertal suppression onto gender-affirming hormones such as estrogen or testosterone would impair fertility. However, this risk has not yet been clearly documented.

† GnRH analogs (puberty blockers) also come as long-acting injections that can last for months, depending on the specific formulation.

just under Meredith's skin, clicked the button to release the implant there, then pulled the device back out. Dr. Stenton covered the cut from the procedure with a small sticker called a Steri-Strip to pull the skin together and let it heal. With that, the procedure was over. The whole thing took less than ten minutes.

It was obviously too early for the implant to have done anything, but Meredith started crying immediately.

Suzanne looked alarmed. "What's wrong, honey!? Is everything okay? Does it hurt?"

"I'm so relieved," Meredith said through her smile, as tears rolled down her blushing cheeks.

6

Choosing Puberty

Estrogen & Testosterone

After pubertal suppression, the next gender-affirming medical interventions adolescents and their families may consider are so-called gender-affirming hormones (estrogen or testosterone), which can initiate a puberty that aligns with the person's gender identity. This chapter will walk you through these medications and how adolescents and their families make decisions about whether they are right for them.

MEREDITH

The next day after having her puberty blocker placed, twelve-year-old Meredith was back in school. The relief she felt was incredible. She remembers sitting in homeroom and her entire body feeling lighter than usual. She held back a smile while she filled out her light pink planner with her schedule for the day, before making small talk with her friends.

When she got home that night, she curled up on the couch in the family room with her mom, dad, and brother to watch a movie. As Meredith was throwing popcorn into her brother's mouth and giggling each time it hit him in the nose, her mom asked her how her day was.

"Honestly—I felt so good." She felt less anxious, more comfortable with herself. With the constant dread of puberty gone, she could live her normal life. For the first time in a while, she was able to just be a kid and focus on schoolwork, her friends, and rehearsals for the school musical that year: *Little Shop of Horrors*. She had landed the role of Audrey—the female lead and love interest of the male lead, Seymour, who adopts a human-eating plant.

"I feel so much better about the show—I can't imagine what it would have been like if my voice started changing while I was singing. I would be humiliated," Meredith pointed out—referencing that without the blocker, testosterone would have thickened and lengthened her vocal cords, causing her voice to crack as it irreversibly deepened.

Ultimately, the show went off without a hitch. She belted out her big song, "Suddenly, Seymour," with a big round of applause from the audience in the school auditorium. Suzanne brought Meredith flowers on opening night. She cradled them with a sheepish grin glowing through her stage makeup.

Over the next year, Meredith lived life like any other middle school girl (albeit an overachieving and type A middle school girl). She had good grades, continued her singing lessons, spent time with friends at the mall, and teased her brother (in child psychiatry we consider this last one a healthy, albeit frustrating for parents, developmental milestone).

But then her classmates began going through puberty. One at a time, her friends would shoot up in height and develop breasts. Friends were talking about bras and periods. Some boys grew facial hair, and their voices started cracking. Meredith felt out of place. Because of her puberty blocker, she was the only student in her class not developing.

She desperately wanted to take estrogen so that she could be on the same timeline as her peers. She didn't want to be the one prepubertal child in her class of developing adolescents. But the Endocrine Society guidelines at the time said that transgender youth generally shouldn't start estrogen until age sixteen.

The reasoning for this came back to a central concern within pediatric gender medicine: doctors were nervous that teenagers would begin hormones, some of the changes from which are irreversible, then change their mind and regret it. As Dr. Forcier explained in the previous chapter, the logic in the earlier years of gender medicine was dominated by the philosophy of "it's better to do nothing and cause harm than to do something and cause harm." The problem was that doing nothing seemed to be causing more and more harm as teens faced untreated gender dysphoria.

For Meredith, she was being forced to sit in a prepubertal stage and deal with the social stress of all her friends developing. She was also falling behind on bone density. Dr. Stenton was tracking it with DEXA scans, and the risk of a bone fracture was still extraordinarily low, but it raised the question: Why did she need to wait until she was sixteen to start estrogen? Did they really think that after all these years she was going to end up identifying as a boy and regret her gender-affirming treatment? Meredith and her family found this preposterous.

When Meredith was fifteen, the family brought this up with Dr. Stenton. She thought they made a lot of sense. In fact, it wasn't the first time she had heard something like this. While the 2009 Endocrine Society guidelines said to wait until sixteen to begin gender-affirming hormones such as estrogen or testosterone, the new 2017 guidelines (which had come out just the year prior) pointed out that, though there weren't as many data about prescribing earlier, there could be compelling reasons to start, sometimes around age fourteen. And those compelling reasons were exactly the ones Meredith was pointing to—bone density concerns and the social stress of having to go through puberty later than peers.

Dr. Stenton ordered some labs to check Meredith's hormone levels and said they could discuss medication more once the labs came back. In preparation for eventually taking estrogen, Meredith and her mom had already had extensive conversations with Dr. Carey and Dr. Stenton, learning a ton about the medication and what would happen if Meredith took it.

Estradiol is considered to be the major "female" sex hormone. By hormone standards, it's a tiny molecule. It's so small, in fact, that it sneaks through the membranes that surround our cells and binds to receptors *inside* the cell.* Those

---

* More recently, researchers have identified that there are also estrogen receptors on the outside of the cell membrane, causing another set of biological reactions. More reading on this is available in this book's endnotes.

estrogen-receptor complexes then move to the nucleus, where our DNA lives, and tell the DNA to make certain proteins, which ultimately result in a range of biological effects, including the physical changes that come with estrogen puberty.

You'll notice that I've been using the word *our* when I talk about estrogen. That's because estrogen isn't only made by people assigned female at birth. Though people generally think of the estrogen created by the ovaries, testes also create estrogen. Additionally, most people assigned male at birth have enzymes in their fat and other tissues that convert testosterone into estrogen. This estrogen is important for a range of physiological processes ranging from bone development to sperm production. While some people think of estrogen for trans women as some sort of "foreign" chemical, gender-affirming hormones are just increasing the levels of a hormone that's already there. The same is true when it comes to testosterone for trans men. In fact, people assigned female at birth have higher levels of testosterone than they do estrogen in their bloodstreams at baseline. Sadly, even many physicians don't realize this, since lab reports use different units for estrogen and testosterone levels. If you ever have sex hormones checked by a lab, you'll notice that testosterone levels are reported in nanograms per deciliter (ng/dL), and estrogen levels are reported in picograms per milliliter (pg/mL).

Prior to starting estrogen, Meredith's doctors showed her a table from the Endocrine Society guidelines that reviewed all the physical changes that come from estrogen, when they start, and when they reach their maximum. Meredith was most surprised (and frustrated) by how long many of the effects would take. Dr. Stenton, however, reminded her that the timeline was similar to what her cisgender peers experience with puberty.

PHYSICAL EFFECTS FROM ESTRADIOL (ESTROGEN)

Effect	Onset	Maximum
Redistribution of body fat	3–6 months	2–3 years
Decrease in muscle mass and strength	3–6 months	1–2 years
Softening of skin and decreased oiliness	3–4 months	Unknown
Decreased sexual desire*	1–3 months	3–6 months
Decreased spontaneous erections	1–3 months	3–6 months
Sexual dysfunction*	Variable	Variable
Breast growth	3–6 months	2–3 years
Decreased testicular volume	3–6 months	2–3 years
Decreased sperm production	Unknown	>3 years
Decreased hair growth†	6–12 months	>3 years
Voice changes	None	None

Meredith learned that estrogen would result in her fat being redistributed in a more "female" rather than a more "male" pattern. This meant more fat in the hip area, for instance,

---

* As I discuss in this chapter, research shows that sexual function generally improves following gender-affirming medical care; however, there are reports of decreased spontaneous erections with use of estradiol.

† While this effect is real, most people who have undergone a testosterone-driven puberty will, depending on their goals, often need other hair-removal strategies such as electrolysis.

along with the development of breast tissue and its accompanying fat. Chest growth, however, is highly variable, and some trans women are disappointed to hear that estrogen results in less chest growth than they may wish. In one study from the Netherlands of 229 trans women taking estrogen, only 11 percent attained an A cup or larger bra size after one year of estrogen therapy. An additional study of 69 trans women by the same research team found that, after three years on estrogen, 29 percent had achieved an A cup or larger. Of note, however, the second study also found that 58 percent of trans women were satisfied with their degree of breast development after treatment. This is in contrast with studies of cis women showing that only about one-quarter are satisfied with their breast development. While there have been anecdotal reports that supplementing estrogen treatment with progesterone may increase the degree of breast development, there is limited concrete evidence this is effective. I should also mention that many trans women anecdotally report much more breast development with estrogen and believe the medical literature underestimates the amount of chest growth that can occur over longer periods of time.

Other generally favorable effects from estrogen include softening of skin and a decrease in skin oiliness, which can sometimes improve acne. While there can be some decrease in hair growth, this tends not to be absolute, and for trans people who have had the effects of testosterone puberty in their system for a substantial period of time, they often, depending on their goals, also need to undergo electrolysis or laser treatment to eliminate unwanted hair growth. On the flip side, estrogen treatment decreases the likelihood of "male"-pattern balding—a type of balding that comes from testosterone and involves loss of hair at the temples and on the top of the head.

Because voice changes primarily come from the thickening and lengthening of vocal cords from testosterone, estrogen treatment doesn't have a substantial impact on voice (it cannot undo the physical changes to the vocal cords from testosterone puberty). For Meredith, though, having been spared testosterone puberty, this was less of an issue. For trans women who do go through testosterone puberty, speech and language pathologists can offer specialized voice training to help them modulate their voice. Vocal cord surgeries are also an option for adults, but currently their results are somewhat unpredictable.

The Endocrine Society guidelines have a comment that estrogen will cause a decrease in muscle mass and strength. Generally, this means something more akin to having a typical "female" musculature rather than more clinically dangerous "muscle wasting." Furthermore, the research in this regard is mixed and remains controversial, particularly when it comes to athletic performance and sports participation, something we'll discuss later.

Another somewhat confusing part of the guidelines is their discussion of sexual functioning following estrogen treatment. It's certainly true that estrogen can result in a decrease in spontaneous erections, something that can be a welcome change for the many trans women who are distressed by their genitalia. But the cited "decrease in sexual desire" is more complex than the guidelines let on.

What's neglected here is that for many trans people, physical gender dysphoria can make sex and intimacy extraordinarily difficult, and at times traumatic. But once they start gender-affirming medical care and their bodies begin to align more with whom they know themselves to be, they feel more self-assured and comfortable, making romance, sex, and intimacy easier.

In 2020, researchers from Amsterdam published a study in the journal *Pediatrics*, looking at the impact of gender-affirming hormones on sexual and romantic development among transgender teens and young adults. The study included 113 young adults who had received puberty blockers, gender-affirming hormones (estrogen or testosterone), and eventually gender-affirming surgery as adults. The researchers found that following these gender-affirming treatments, the study participants reported a statistically significant increase in all types of sexual activities examined—both masturbation (suggesting an improvement in their comfort with their own bodies when alone) and sexual behavior with a partner (suggesting increased confidence expressing intimacy with others, likely due to feeling more comfortable in their bodies). For the young adults, sexual intercourse increased from 16.2 percent before surgery to 37.6 percent after surgery.

Meredith herself was starting to have more interest in dating, particularly as several boys in her class had been asking her out on dates. But she still felt too self-conscious and was avoiding it.

Suzanne also found herself in the uncomfortable position of needing to talk to Meredith about balancing privacy regarding her gender history and her safety. The reality was that trans women are often victims of violence, and many of these instances of violence have arisen in the context of intimate partners. Suzanne explained to Meredith that while generally her gender history is personal and no one else's business, that for safety reasons this is something to consider discussing with partners prior to reaching deeper levels of intimacy.

Though transgender bodies are woefully stigmatized in many places today, and people's discomfort even sometimes leads to horrific violence, I remain hopeful that this won't be true for future generations. From working with today's young people, who are much more comfortable around gender diversity and diverse bodies, I think there's reason for hope. Meredith, for example, was out at school, and it was not an issue. Her classmates accepted her, and she had the same classroom romance dramas as the other kids in class.

As many young people do, she went back and forth about how open she wanted to be with her peers when she went off to college. On the one hand, she was proud of her trans identity and saw value in being open. But on the other hand, she recognized it would be easier to just live her life as a girl and not need to talk about it until she was in a situation where it was relevant (perhaps in a romantic relationship where sex and future families were being discussed, or in doctors' appointments). It's something she continued to think about.

The topic does, however, raise another sad reality for many trans kids in the United States. When I spoke with Suzanne alone, she shared with me that she feels lucky Meredith has grown up in an environment that's so liberal and accepting. To her knowledge, Meredith hadn't really experienced overt transphobia. But as Suzanne thought about Meredith's growing up and potentially going off to college, Suzanne suspected her daughter's options might be much more limited because of safety concerns. Would it be safe for Meredith to go to college in the South? Or in a more rural town?* Suzanne was somewhat reassured because she thought both Meredith and her brother were most likely to want to live on one of the coasts anyway—given their academic and professional interests. But the fact that her daughter was limited by something Suzanne couldn't control still broke her heart.

Discussions around starting estrogen also meant revisiting the question of fertility preservation. Meredith and her family had discussed it many times since she had her puberty blocker placed, and a few more questions came up. Meredith was sure she was attracted to men, but what would happen if she ended up dating a trans man who had preserved eggs? If that happened, would they want to have biological children? Meredith thought it was possible, but the prospect of progressing through male puberty to provide a semen sample was just too distressing. Though there were some experimental technologies available to take a biopsy of testicular tissue and potentially use it to create sperm in the future, she didn't want to undergo this invasive procedure. She and her family also talked about the many ways to build a family—including through adoption—all of which were valid. She and her family ultimately decided to forgo fertility preservation and proceed with estrogen.

In the appointment with Dr. Stenton to review the estrogen consent forms, Meredith's family reviewed all the risks, benefits, and potential side effects again. Generally, estrogen is very well tolerated when used in gender-affirming medical care. But

---

* As an aside, I shared with Suzanne here that I had heard from my colleagues who study the mental health of trans youth in rural communities that many of these communities actually rally around trans kids. These smaller communities, though often steeped in traditional values, are also close-knit, and when a young person needs something, people are there to provide love, support, and protection in any way that a kid needs.

doctors always still review a few things. Research from estrogen-containing oral contraceptive pills suggests that estrogen may increase the risk of a blood clot. Based on the data we have so far, it still appears to be very rare for someone to develop a blood clot from estrogen when used for gender-affirming medical care. It's more likely if someone has an underlying genetic blood-clotting disorder, so doctors always take a careful family history of any blood clots in the legs, lungs, or brain.* It's also more likely if someone smokes cigarettes, which we always counsel patients to avoid, but especially if they're taking estrogen. When Dr. Stenton brought this up, Meredith scrunched up her nose, saying, "That's disgusting." Luckily, this disgust toward cigarettes is something we're hearing from younger generations more and more lately. Lastly, some trans women wish to see the physical effects of estrogen more quickly and may take higher doses of estrogen than recommended, sometimes even buying the medication online. If levels get too high from this, people are again at risk of a serious blood clot. Dr. Stenton reviewed with Meredith that taking higher-than-recommended doses generally increases the risk of blood clots without having much additional impact on physical development.

They also discussed the impact of taking estrogen on future cancer screenings that would occur well into adulthood. Because data are somewhat limited regarding the optimal cancer screenings, doctors recommend that people have cancer screenings

---

* There are some ways to potentially mitigate the risk of blood clots for those with underlying clotting conditions who wish to start estrogen, including using estrogen patches instead of pills, and ensuring that the underlying clotting condition is adequately treated, when relevant.

both for any organ they have, and for any organ relevant to the hormone they are taking. For instance, because Meredith still had a prostate, she should follow the usual prostate cancer screenings written for cisgender men once she reached adulthood. And because she would be taking estrogen, she should, as an adult, have the same routine breast cancer screenings as cisgender women (though the risk of breast cancer is still *much* lower among trans women than it is among cis women). Similarly, a trans man taking testosterone should continue having cervical cancer screenings if he still has a cervix.*

With all of those discussions completed, Dr. Stenton sent an electronic prescription for estradiol pills (the most commonly used form of estrogen) to the pharmacy, and Meredith and Suzanne went to pick it up.† While there are other forms of estrogen available, including a patch (more expensive but with a lower risk of blood clots for people who have a concerning blood-clotting history), Meredith thought the pill would be easiest.

They stopped by Walgreens to get the pills right after the appointment, then returned back home. Meredith couldn't

---

* Sadly, many trans men are hesitant to visit a gynecologist to have this done, as their practices aren't always affirming of trans men. This continues to be a major issue today. However, younger generations of physicians are becoming more interested in setting up practices that are affirming of trans men and nonbinary people and their health care needs.

† People taking gender-affirming estrogen usually need a second medication to suppress their endogenous testosterone production. Because Meredith had her puberty blocker in place, she didn't need an additional medication. Others who don't have a puberty blocker in place may take another medication called spironolactone to block their testosterone production. People taking testosterone generally don't need a second medication, as testosterone effectively suppresses estrogen production on its own.

wait to take her first dose and took it that night. Even though it would take a long time before there would be any physical effects, just taking the pill gave her an overwhelming feeling of comfort and peace. She felt like herself.

SAM

Around the same time, Sam, who was still using any pronouns (*he*, *she*, and *they*, depending on the day), was also starting to have thoughts about puberty. She and her mom had been talking about it a lot. Kate had picked up a few child-friendly books about puberty from the bookstore, and they went through them together.

In a meeting I had with Kate, she looked at me and shrugged. "He says he doesn't care; either puberty sounds fine to him." She told me that they had met with their endocrinologist, who recently confirmed Sam had entered the early stages of testosterone puberty. Sam told her that he wasn't interested in a puberty blocker. He continued to identify as sometimes a girl and sometimes a boy and was moving between different pronouns depending on the given day and his gender feelings.

Like many kids I work with, Sam had settled into a nonbinary gender identity. This includes a wide range of gender identities that are neither strictly male nor strictly female. Though Sam didn't ascribe a particular label to his gender identity, some people whose gender identity fluctuates between male and female identify as *gender fluid*, highlighting the dynamic (or fluid) nature of how they experience or ascribe language to their gender identity, and sometimes their gender expression as well.

Nonbinary youth will sometimes still have physical gender dysphoria and desire medical interventions like puberty blockers to alleviate this distress. But Sam felt okay with his body and was comfortable going through testosterone puberty. He would change his gender expression on different days (a dress one day and using *she* pronouns, and gym shorts and using *he* pronouns another day). For him, the gender expression was important for feeling like his authentic self, but the physical development of his body didn't feel as important. He was aware that the physical changes of male puberty would be essentially permanent, and he felt okay with this. The treatment team and his mother asked him to keep them updated if things ever changed (in the same way that we regularly check in with kids undergoing puberty from exogenous hormones to see if their desires ever change).

Some nonbinary youth with physical gender dysphoria undergo the usual treatments like those Meredith had. But others will choose to take very low doses of estrogen or testosterone to induce lesser levels of masculinization or feminization than the standard doses generally preferred by adolescents with binary gender identities. In the same way that there are many different gender identities and many ways to be trans, there's a wide range of physical gendered manifestations that make people feel comfortable.* But again, Sam felt comfortable without any medical intervention.

---

* Some nonbinary youth experience distress at the prospect of both male and female puberty. They sometimes wish they could stay on pubertal suppression indefinitely. Unfortunately, this would not be safe for bone health. Though some have highlighted that medications called selective estrogen receptor modulators (SERMs) could potentially mineralize the bones without causing other unwanted physical effects for nonbinary youth, these haven't yet been tested and aren't in clinical use (see Pang et al., "Long-Term Puberty Suppression," in this book's endnotes).

For Sam, puberty ended up going off without a hitch. And beautifully, his community rallied around him. He felt most comfortable using the gender-neutral bathroom at school, which the administration facilitated. His friends remained mostly girls, and they welcomed him with open arms. He had regular playdates throughout the week and joined the school's coed soccer team. When his English class put on a short play for a school project and he gravitated to a female role, the teacher let him play the part he wanted.

All the while, Sam's self-confidence and mental health continued to flourish. He was a happy healthy kid and was blossoming into a confident adolescent. His development was a sharp contrast with other kids I had seen who were forced into gender boxes, or bullied and harassed for their gender nonconformity.

Sam's story is an important reminder to us that gender is complex and different for everyone. People's gender identities and expressions don't always fit into the neat binary boxes we expect. Some people desire medical interventions and absolutely need them, and others don't want them but still identify under the trans umbrella. The important thing is that we listen to kids and let them be themselves. When we do, they thrive.

KYLE

After I met Kyle in the emergency room, he was transferred to an inpatient psychiatric hospital to stabilize his mental health and get him to a psychological state in which he would be safe to go home again.

He had mixed feelings about the hospital stay. On the one hand, it was miserable. Because of their safety protocols, the staff took away his shoelaces, and he wasn't allowed to have his cell phone. It all felt dehumanizing. He also had to sleep there overnight with a roommate, away from the comfort of home.

But there were also some good things that happened while he was there. The hospital had a policy of rooming people based on their gender identity, so Kyle ended up having a male room-mate, something that made him feel affirmed and respected in a way he hadn't before.*

The therapist on the unit also had a series of meetings with him and his parents, in which Kyle was finally able to have open conversations about his gender dysphoria and the way it made him feel.

Rosa and Juan felt awful about how Kyle had been suffering, and it was difficult for them to hear that their early attempts to push him to identify as a girl, motivated by their wanting to protect him, had caused him intense shame. It was a lot for them to take in, and they still struggled to fully understand, but those early conversations in the hospital opened up a line of commu-nication between Kyle and his parents to start talking about it more, and his parents committed to ongoing conversations.

Hearing that his parents were open to talking about his gender, and even open to using the name Kyle and *he* pro-nouns when they went home, gave Kyle immense hope. By the time he left the hospital, his suicidal thoughts had dramatically improved. Though he was still stressed by his gender dysphoria,

---

* For mental-health-care workers reading this, we recently published an article on how to make inpatient psychiatric facilities more comfortable for transgender and gender-diverse youth (see Acosta et al., "Identify, Engage, Understand," in this book's endnotes).

this new open line of conversation with his parents helped him see a path forward in which he could be himself, while getting love and support. His parents signed up to go to a support group for the parents of trans kids, so that they could process what was going on and learn more. They were still skeptical of the notion of Kyle's starting testosterone, which he had voiced an interest in, but they worked with the inpatient team to set him up with an outpatient therapist to talk to about everything that was impacting his mental health: his depression, his eating disorder symptoms, and his gender. The inpatient team also set the family up with a family therapist to help them work on keeping these conversations going. Kyle tended to shut down when he felt ashamed, and his parents tended to want to avoid conversations about gender, which made them feel nervous and out of their depth. The family therapist would help them push through these avoidance urges and bring them closer together both emotionally and in terms of their understanding of how to support any gender-related needs Kyle might have.

When they got back home, Kyle began meeting with a therapist named Andrés. They went through a similar process to the one Meredith went through with Dr. Carey, exploring all the facets of Kyle's gender history, his eating disorder symptoms (which seemed almost entirely driven by his gender dysphoria),* and his depression. Over time, it became clear to Andrés and Kyle that most of his difficulties were stemming from his

---

* Though this was the case for Kyle, eating disorder symptoms can be diverse among trans youth. Sometimes they are driven entirely by gender dysphoria. Sometimes they aren't driven by gender dysphoria at all. Often the two become intermingled in a way that is difficult to tease apart, or the eating disorder symptoms may start from gender dysphoria and later take on a life of their own.

physical gender dysphoria and that it needed to be addressed. Andrés talked to Kyle more about testosterone—what it does, what it doesn't do, and any potential side effects. Andrés also started to introduce this information to Kyle's parents early on, encouraging them to read materials made by the University of California, San Francisco, which educate patients and families about how testosterone hormone therapy works.*

While Kyle was going through his own personal therapy, his parents also began attending the local support group for the parents of trans youth. Having read a great deal of negative information about trans youth in the media, they entered the group skeptical. They were particularly wary of some of the physicians who worked in gender-affirming medical care, as they had read in conservative news outlets that these doctors were biased and not practicing best care.† But hearing from other parents who had gone through a similar journey changed things for them. Sitting on folding chairs in a local high school

---

* I often recommend this website from UCSF as initial reading for families to understand testosterone treatment and how it works: Madeline Deutsch, "Overview of Masculinizing Hormone Therapy," https://transcare.ucsf.edu/article/information-testosterone-hormone-therapy.

† This has been a sad reality in the news in recent years, where there is commonly misinformation spread about trans youth and their health care. For instance, many right-wing outlets advocate for legislative bans on gender-affirming medical care for trans adolescents, despite every major medical organization, including the American Medical Association, the American Academy of Pediatrics, the American Psychiatric Association, and the American Academy of Child & Adolescent Psychiatry, opposing such legislation. For a summary and list of statements from major medical organizations, see Turban, Kraschel, and Cohen, "Legislation to Criminalize Gender-Affirming Medical Care for Transgender Youth" in this book's endnotes.

gym, they heard from actual parents who had also gone from skeptical of affirming their children's gender identity to watching them thrive once they were supported and affirmed. Many parents lamented that gender-affirming medical care couldn't fix everything (transphobia, bullying, other mental health conditions such as major depressive disorder), but it had dramatic positive impacts for their kids, whom the parents saw as more confident and comfortable in their bodies.

These parents were also able to talk to Rosa and Juan about some of the common experiences parents of trans youth have when their children come out.* Many of these parents were worried that their children's gender identity was a phase and that they would start hormones and later regret them. The parents were able to tell Rosa and Juan that they understood their reservations; every parent wants the best future for their child and feels responsible for their decisions, especially medical ones. But the parents also helped Rosa and Juan broaden their minds to consider not just the risks of allowing Kyle to take testosterone, but also what would happen if he didn't. The reality is that they would never know with 100 percent certainty which was the right path forward (testosterone or no testosterone), but they needed to fully weigh the risks and benefits of either path. Rosa and Juan reflected more on how Kyle's gender dysphoria had been hurting him—especially his

---

* I always tell parents it's essential they have a place to talk through things without their children present. I've treated many transgender adults for whom something their parents said in passing stuck in their mind and impacted their self-esteem for a lifetime. It wasn't the parents' final thought, or something they truly deeply believed, but the passing comment made a dramatic negative impact. It's vital families have a safe space to be validated and organize their thoughts on gender before bringing their thoughts to their children.

eating disorder symptoms—and started to wonder how things would be different if he took testosterone. The standard treatments they had tried for anorexia didn't work—maybe it truly was because the gender dysphoria was the problem.

One of the other parents also brought up that his son struggled a lot with distress related to periods and that an oral contraceptive pill called Aygestin* had helped stop his periods and provided relief. This seemed like a no-brainer since so many cisgender girls took oral contraceptive pills anyway. Rosa and Juan talked to Kyle's primary-care doctor, who prescribed this for him right away. It was a huge help for Kyle. Though not a magic cure for his eating disorder symptoms because he still worried about chest development, he did start eating more once he was on the pill and felt reassured his periods would be suppressed. And he told Andrés that each time he took it, it was a warm reminder that his parents were supporting and understanding him more.

Rosa and Juan were also able to talk to the other parents about how they felt a strong connection to Kyle's birth name and the ideas they had around what his life would be like as an adult. How could they let go of those dreams they had and the name they had so carefully chosen?

One of the other parents, a burly truck driver named Bruce, who had a trans daughter, yelled out gruffly, "Your kids never grow up the way you expect! That's normal! Ain't nothing special about trans kids there!"

---

* Aygestin is a popular oral contraceptive pill used in gender care because it does not contain estrogen. Though estrogen-containing oral contraceptive pills are also effective, many trans masculine people feel more psychologically comfortable with a medication that doesn't contain estrogen.

Everyone let out a laugh, but it was a bit of an aha moment for Rosa and Juan. Why were they so caught up in this vision they had about Kyle's life? Of course kids never grow up exactly the way parents expect. What was important was that they find a path forward to make sure he thrived as well as he could. Harkening back to the work of psychologist Dr. Alison Gopnik and the carpenter-versus-gardener approaches to parenting, Rosa and Juan were starting to think more about how they could cultivate rather than try to shape their child.

After about a year of discussions in the parent support group, family therapy, and Kyle working in his individual therapy, Kyle and his parents met with an adolescent-medicine doctor at a gender clinic about an hour away from their house. It was a long drive in the heat, and everyone was nervous.

Sitting in an exam room, the endocrinologist taught the family a bit more about testosterone (though in reality they knew most of it, having had long conversations with Kyle's therapist and having read through the UCSF materials in detail). They went through a table similar to that Meredith went through for estrogen, also from the Endocrine Society guidelines.

Most of these didn't come as a surprise. The family knew about the risk of worsening acne, that facial hair would develop and be mostly irreversible with time, and that body fat would redistribute to a male pattern. Opposite to the effect of Meredith's estrogen treatment, Kyle would be *more likely* to develop "male"-pattern hair loss on his head. Unlike estrogen though, testosterone would have a substantial impact on voice—deepening the pitch as the vocal cords thickened and lengthened. Luckily, the family had already had a difficult therapy

PHYSICAL EFFECTS OF TESTOSTERONE

Effect	Onset	Maximum
Increase in skin oiliness and acne	1–6 months	1–2 years
Facial and body hair growth	6–12 months	4–5 years
Scalp hair loss	6–12 months	Unknown
Increased muscle mass/strength	6–12 months	2–5 years
Fat redistribution	1–6 months	2–5 years
Cessation of menses (periods)	1–6 months	Unknown
Clitoral enlargement	1–6 months	1–2 years
Vaginal atrophy	1–6 months	1–2 years
Voice deepening	6–12 months	1–2 years

session in which they'd talked about the realities of Kyle's clitoris growing from testosterone and the risk of vaginal atrophy.* They had also had extensive conversations about fertility preservation. Though they were interested in it, they simply could not afford it, something that weighed heavily into their calculus around starting the medication.

They also spoke about the different ways testosterone could be given. The most common way is by a self-administered injection, since it tends to give fairly consistent dosing. There's also a gel available, but it can be inconvenient, since it takes time to dry, and you need to be careful not to accidentally get it on

---

* A condition that can be painful but can also be treated with topical estrogen creams, which aren't absorbed much into the bloodstream and thus don't negatively impact testosterone therapy.

other people before it does. Patches were available as well, but could causes rashes and weren't popular. Though his parents weren't ready for Kyle to start yet, he said he'd most likely go with the injections if things moved forward. This surprised Rosa and Juan, since Kyle had always been horrified of needles. It had once taken three people to hold him down at the pediatrician's office to get his vaccines. Kyle's parents took a mental note of the moment as a reminder of how important this must be to him.

About a month after the appointment, Kyle sat his parents down in the living room. "Why are we still waiting?" he asked, his voice shaking. "It's been a year, and I've answered all your questions; I've been in therapy this whole time. I just don't get it. I know you're nervous about me changing my mind. I can't promise you I never will, but I can tell you that I think it's really unlikely. I can't predict the future, but I can tell you how badly I want this *now* and have for so long. What more do I need to do?"

Rosa and Juan didn't have an answer. Kyle looked his mom straight in the eyes, as his own began to well up with tears.

"Okay. Dad and I will talk about it tonight, and we'll all talk about it again tomorrow."

Kyle accepted their answer and went to bed early.

That night, Rosa and Juan stayed up late in bed going through the binder of materials they had collected about gender dysphoria and testosterone. Juan turned to Rosa and pointed out that it *had* been a really long time that they'd been discussing this, and Kyle had been struggling for years. Was testosterone really scarier than what they had been going through with his depression and eating disorder? It was starting to feel as if they were hurting their child—the image of his tear-filled eyes from earlier that night continued popping into Rosa's mind. They finally decided together that they would tell him the next day that they would take him to get the testosterone prescription. And they'd watch closely to see how he responded. It would take at least a month on the medication before any obvious physical changes took place, and they could see how things went. The endocrinologist and Andrés always reminded them that they would check in with Kyle regularly and that he could stop the testosterone at any time. It was time to give it a go.

The next morning, when Kyle came down for breakfast, Juan was filling everyone's bright yellow bowls with Frosted Flakes and pouring glasses of orange juice.

"Well, this is nice . . . ," Kyle said, used to them just grabbing their own breakfasts from the cabinets in the morning.

Rosa motioned for him to sit down, and she and Juan sat at the opposite side of the walnut table, a long lace runner dividing either side. "We're going to call the clinic today for the testosterone. Andrés has already sent in the letter, and they have your labs on file, so they should be able to send in the prescription and set up a time for you to go in and learn how to do the injections." They had also already gone through and signed the informed consent forms with the doctor at the last appointment, in case they decided to start.

Kyle's eyebrows furrowed while a small smile formed at the edge of his right lip—a facial expression that combined skepticism and excitement.

Rosa's and Juan's faces looked concerned. "Is everything okay?"

"There are just so many emotions going on—I'm so excited to be starting, and so sad about everything I've gone through; it's just a lot." After a few minutes, Kyle calmed down and thanked his parents, telling them that it really meant a lot to him. They called the clinic and left a message for the doctor.

They got a message back through the online patient portal that the testosterone prescription had been sent to the pharmacy and that they had an appointment with the nurse in two days for her to teach them how to do the injections.

They drove to CVS to pick up the prescription, and Rosa said she would hold on to it until they had the appointment because the needles made her nervous. Kyle sat in the back seat of the car sipping on an iced tea that they'd also picked up at CVS, a big smile on his face as they drove home.

On the day of the appointment to learn how to do his injections, all three packed into the car and set off for the hour-long drive back to the clinic. Juan asked how Kyle was feeling, and he said it was a weird combination of nervous and excited. He felt a ton of butterflies dancing all around in his stomach.

They made it to the clinic on time, and the medical assistant brought them back into an exam room. The nurse came in and asked them if they were ready, and Kyle nodded yes. The nurse explained that the easiest place to do the testosterone injection was on the belly, but that they'd first need to prepare the syringe.

The nurse had Kyle wash his hands and showed him how to take the cap off the vial of medication and clean the top with an alcohol swab. He held the plastic syringe in his hand, and she showed him how to attach the needle so he could draw the medication from the vial into the syringe. She then took the big needle (for drawing up medication) off the syringe and put on the much smaller needle used for the actual injection. He laughed with relief to know that the one he actually did the injection with was much smaller.

But overall, his parents were shocked that he was managing all this needle business so easily. Rosa said, "How are you handling this so well?"

Kyle turned and said, "Mom, I've been waiting for this for over a year—I'm not thinking about the needles!"

Kyle lifted up the bottom of his hoodie, cleaned the belly area with an alcohol swab the way the nurse instructed, then quickly did the injection. "That was easy."

The nurse reminded him to not always inject in the same exact place, since some people say that can cause hair growth on the skin at that area, a comment that made Kyle giggle before he said he definitely would not forget that.

Like Meredith, Kyle felt a wave of excitement and relief, though he knew it would still take a while for the testosterone to cause obvious physical effects. Juan and Rosa were surprised by how anticlimactic the whole thing felt—it was such an easy procedure, and they were already on the drive back home.

They picked up a pizza on the way back, then sat around the table for dinner. It felt as if they were back to their normal life, like a large gray cloud had lifted up and away from the table. Kyle was smiling and talking about how he was excited to go to school the next year, and he asked them if they wanted to watch a movie that night. They smiled and told him they'd love to.

7

Gender Surgery

Talking about gender makes many people uncomfortable, and talking about surgery makes many people scared. This chapter nonetheless tackles the topic of gender surgery. I'll discuss some of the most common surgeries that transgender people consider, including gender-affirming mastectomy (removal of chest tissue for people assigned female at birth) and gender-affirming vaginoplasty (surgical construction of a vagina).*

---

* There are a range of other gender-affirming surgeries that are considered for adults. So many, in fact, that discussing them all is outside the scope of this book. Some are briefly mentioned in the appendices. They include gender-affirming facial surgery (a major surgery to undo the impacts of testosterone puberty on the facial bones), breast augmentation, phalloplasty (construction of a penis), and thyroid chondroplasty (removal of the Adam's apple), among others. All of these are highly individualized procedures and at the time of this writing are generally not performed on minors. As gender surgeons are quick to note, early medical intervention with pubertal suppression can make many of these

Under current medical guidelines, gender-affirming genital surgeries are generally reserved for adults.* I talk about them here so that parents and readers can know what may be down the line for young trans people later in life. It is likely that surgical techniques will continue to evolve over time, and for that reason, the content of this chapter may become outdated by the time you read it. It is essential that anyone considering surgery speak directly with a surgeon, both because these techniques are constantly evolving over time, and because specific practices may vary surgeon by surgeon. Nonetheless, I hope this chapter will provide a general sense of the important considerations regarding gender-affirming surgery. Finally, this chapter has some detailed descriptions of surgical techniques that could bother the squeamish. Please make sure you're in a comfortable headspace before reading, if you fall into that category.

KYLE

For the first few weeks after starting testosterone, Kyle didn't notice very much, other than his mood being better. Now that

---

surgeries (e.g., gender-affirming top surgery, gender-affirming facial surgery, and body contouring), many of which can be quite intensive, unnecessary. This is an important aspect of weighing risks and benefits of starting pubertal suppression during adolescence.

* This has historically been the case and is currently the case with the latest Endocrine Society guidelines. The most recent WPATH Standards of Care removed age cutoffs for surgeries, but I suspect most surgeons will interpret this, given the past guidelines, as still reserving genital surgeries for adults and will consider younger ages only in very specific circumstances (e.g., a seventeen-year-old who wishes to have a vaginoplasty in the summer before college, to prevent needing to recover during the academic semester).

he had hope that his body would start to match who he was, he felt a major sense of relief.

By six months of taking testosterone, he was noticing some effects. His voice started to first crack, then eventually deepen. He grew more body hair, including on his abdomen. There was less fat on his hips, and he noticed his musculature was looking more toned. But one thing didn't change at all—his chest. He continued to wear his binder to flatten it the best he could, but his chest would still show, even to a degree when wearing loose clothes, and he hated it. It made him not want to go to gym class. It made him not want to go to the beach or to the neighborhood pool with his friends. He still wanted to avoid showers.

Some recent research has shown that although testosterone helps with gender dysphoria, chest dysphoria can worsen for some people, as they feel better about other parts of their body aligning with who they are and begin to focus more on the part that isn't. In a qualitative study published in the journal *Pediatrics* in 2021, one study participant explained, "When I started [testosterone, my chest dysphoria] got worse, because other things that were causing me dysphoria lessened . . . so it made my chest dysphoria feel worse in comparison. . . . It probably was the same, but the fact that everything else, like . . . voice dysphoria was getting a bit better—it made my chest dysphoria more prominent in comparison." The adolescents in that study said that the one thing that helped with their chest dysphoria was having gender-affirming top surgery.

The thought of surgery scared seventeen-year-old Kyle, but his chest dysphoria was also making him miserable. He read more about gender-affirming mastectomy (often called top surgery) online.

He learned that there were a few different types. The first is called a keyhole surgery. In this kind of surgery, the surgeon makes an incision around the areola and removes breast tissue. This is followed by liposuction to contour the chest. As Kyle read more, he learned that this surgery was only an option for people with a very small amount of chest tissue. Because Kyle had gone through so much estrogen puberty and had a fair amount of chest growth, it wasn't an option for him.

Because most trans boys and nonbinary people seeking gender-affirming mastectomy are in Kyle's situation of having gone through estrogen puberty before they can access gender-affirming care,* the vast majority are only candidates for the other common type of top surgery: a double incision procedure. This surgery involves making an incision along the crease under the breast and a second along where the bottom of the pectoralis muscle sits. Chest tissue is then removed, and the skin is sutured back together so that a scar sits along the bottoms of the pectoralis muscles on each side of the chest.[†] The goal of this is to hide the scar along the curve of the pec muscle, though the scar tends to still be quite visible on most people. The surgeon can also remove the nipple and make it smaller and more oval for a more "masculine" nipple aesthetic prior to suturing it back into place. Because the nipple is removed and replaced, there

---

* It's worth noting that for those who access pubertal suppression early, they never develop substantial breast tissue and thus don't need future gender-affirming chest surgery.

† San Francisco gender-affirming surgeon Scott Mosser has created an animated video that gives an overview of the surgery and relevant anatomy: https://youtu .be/zSslDLCrxD8?si=FOmıthRwuvZndooc.

can be permanent loss of sensation of the nipple, though many patients develop feeling again over time.

In a variation of this procedure, called the buttonhole procedure, the surgeon does not remove the nipple. Instead, she leaves a flap of tissue from the bottom of the chest leading up to the nipple and, when closing the tissue, buries that flap inside the chest. She then cuts through the chest to reveal the nipple below and sutures it into place. Because this approach aims to keep the nerve and blood supply to the nipple intact, it hopes to maintain nipple sensation at a higher rate than the general double-incision procedure, though it is not 100 percent successful in maintaining sensation. The surgeon must also carefully assess an individual patient to see if they are a candidate for the approach, based on how the buried flap of tissue would impact chest contour.

As Kyle learned more about top surgery, he realized it would be a big decision. It wasn't a small surgery, and it would require recovery time. Some surgeons leave drains in place following the surgery for any fluid that collects in the chest. He would need to wear a compressive chest binder for a week after surgery and couldn't do any heavy lifting or raise his arms above his head for a month. The surgery also carried potential risks: the loss of nipple sensation, infection, bleeding, and the usual risks of anesthesia. Though the likelihood of these were low, they were still scary. He also read about how different people could end up with different scars—sometimes raised, red, or stretched. Some surgeons' websites explained that there were techniques that could be used—such as tension-reducing clips on the incision closure or certain medications—to reduce the risk of scars looking worse than usual. But Kyle knew that even with the best healing, there would be two large scars.

Kyle brought up with his therapist, Andrés, that he was reading about top surgery and considering asking his parents about
it. Andrés walked through what Kyle had learned online about
top surgery to make sure everything he read was accurate. Andrés
also brought up one thing that Kyle hadn't thought about in a
while: fertility. His family had not been able to afford fertility
preservation for him, so he wasn't sure if he would ultimately be
able to have biological children, though he did think he might
want to one day. Though it was possible that testosterone would
impair his fertility, Andrés pointed out that there were many
instances of people who had started testosterone, then temporarily stopped and had been able to have their own biological
children. Having top surgery would mean that if Kyle went down
this route, he would not be able to chestfeed any child he might
have. It was a weird thing to think about and something that
had never crossed Kyle's mind. He spent the next few weeks in
between his sessions with Andrés thinking about it. The more
he reflected, the more he realized his chest dysphoria would
prevent him from ever being able to chestfeed a child anyway.
The idea of having biological children was still overwhelming,
and he couldn't be sure if he would want to do that or not. But he
was fairly certain he wouldn't want to chestfeed if he did. Even
if he were wrong, he felt confident the improvement in chest
dysphoria he would feel outweighed the risk.

He talked about it with his parents, and his mom told him
for the first time that she herself wasn't able to chestfeed him,
and that he had been given mostly formula, something that made
his mom feel guilty, given what the pediatrician told her about
the benefits of breast milk for an infant. The conversations made
Kyle feel uncomfortable. Many of these talks around the risks of

surgery, chestfeeding, babies, and what surgical recovery would be like overwhelmed him. He decided to table the conversation for a month to clear his mind and digest the information.

Each night when he got in the shower though, he would think about it. When he put his binder on, he would think about it more. When he noticed his chest was still visible under his hoodie, he'd think about it. Despite how scary some things about top surgery seemed, the burden and stress of the chest dysphoria were too much. He wanted to have the surgery. He told his parents and therapist that he needed it, and they agreed to schedule a consultation with a surgeon to at least learn more. To their distress, they learned it would be months before he could get in to see someone for even just a consultation.

On the day the consultation was scheduled, Kyle woke up early—feeling both trepidation and hope. He and his parents drove about forty-five minutes to a nearby surgeon. The nurse called them back to the office, where three chairs sat on one side of the desk, and the surgeon sat on the other. His walls were covered in diplomas.

Kyle had submitted photos ahead of time, which the surgeon had reviewed, and confirmed that Kyle would be a candidate for a double incision procedure. It was up to Kyle and his parents if they wanted to do either the standard nipple grafting or the buttonhole approach. The surgeon thought either would work with Kyle's anatomy.

Over the course of about forty-five minutes, the surgeon walked Kyle and his parents through much of the information they had already gotten about top surgery. The surgeon also showed them before-and-after pictures of patients on whom he had operated. The surgeon spoke seriously about all the risks of surgery and what the recovery would be like. Because Kyle and his parents had waited so long for the appointment, they had pretty much made up their minds. They booked the appointment for the surgery, which, because of the long wait list, wouldn't be for another eight months. During those months, Andrés would check in with Kyle periodically to see if any new thoughts or feelings emerged about having the surgery. Kyle was sure he wanted it.

The morning of surgery, just a month before his eighteenth birthday, Kyle woke up at five in the morning and drove to the surgery center with his parents. They were greeted by a nurse who brought him back to the preoperative area, made sure he was comfortable in a gown and propped up with pillows, and placed an IV in his arm. After a few minutes, the surgeon came in to say hi. He walked Kyle through the steps of the surgery again, then brought him to the operating room, where the team helped him get comfortable on the operating table.

The anesthesiologist told him to take deep breaths while she pushed medication into the IV, and he fell asleep. The next thing he remembered, he was in the postoperative area with his mom and dad standing next to him. He didn't have any pain but was groggy. The surgeon came in, told him everything had gone as expected, and Kyle's parents took him back home to recover, wearing a tight binder.

Later that week, he went back to the surgeon for his first follow-up appointment. Some pain had started once the local anesthesia wore off, but it was manageable with the pain medication from the doctor. The surgeon checked that the incisions were healing well, which they were. During that appointment,

Kyle put on a T-shirt and looked in the mirror. He was beaming. He finally looked like his true self.

The surgeon explained that the recovery would take a while. For the next month, Kyle shouldn't lift more than twenty pounds or lift his arms above his head. This was to make sure the healing went well, and so that his scars didn't stretch. Kyle didn't care. It was finally done.

MEREDITH

Though estrogen made a huge difference for Meredith to feel more comfortable in her body, she still struggled with how she felt about dating. Boys in her high school would regularly ask her out, but her discomfort toward her bottom half made her too self-conscious. She didn't necessarily think she would be sexually active in high school, but she worried about what would happen down the road.

Throughout high school, undistracted by dating and committed to her classes, she continued to get straight A's. She bonded with her close-knit group of friends, all similarly academically minded, who just saw her as another girl. The fact that she was transgender rarely came up. What seemed more relevant was the unspoken competition that permeated their school regarding upcoming college admissions and who would be valedictorian. In her junior year, she sent college applications off—mostly, as her mom had predicted, to schools in New England and California.

As she waited for college admissions decisions, she talked to Dr. Carey more about her feelings regarding a vaginoplasty. She was steadfast in wanting to have it done. She and her mother had already researched surgeons extensively, and they wanted her to have the surgery the summer before she went off to college, so her studies wouldn't be interrupted by the recovery time.

Dr. Carey talked to Meredith about how a vaginoplasty is done, and Meredith learned that it's a big surgery. The most common approach was called an inversion phalloplasty, in which the skin from the penis and scrotum are used to construct the lining of the vaginal canal. However, because Meredith had undergone pubertal suppression at a young age, she didn't have enough skin available to create sufficient vaginal depth. For this reason, she would likely need to undergo a peritoneal pull-through surgery, in which some of the vaginal canal was constructed with the internal lining of the abdomen.*

The recovery from the surgery would be long. She would need to stay in the hospital for a few days postoperatively for monitoring and pain control. She wouldn't be able to start doing light aerobic activity again for around six weeks, no strenuous activity would be allowed for two to three months. She learned that she'd also have to forgo swimming for three months, meaning that she'd miss the summer pool parties some of her friends were planning.

After one undergoes a vaginoplasty, one also needs to regularly "dilate" using progressively larger dilators that keep the vaginal canal open. If she didn't follow this dilation regimen, the vaginal canal would likely scar down and close. For the first three months, she would need to dilate three times per day,

---

* While Meredith and Dr. Carey discussed this specific peritoneal vaginoplasty technique, many people in this situation still undergo a standard penile-inversion vaginoplasty and extend the canal using skin grafts from the abdomen or hips.

with the frequency gradually decreasing over time. Though the frequency decreases, it is generally something one needs to do for life to prevent the vagina from shrinking or closing.

There were also some rare but serious risks of surgery. The one surgeons tend to worry about the most is called a recto-vaginal fistula, in which an opening forms between the newly created vagina and the rectum, leading to fecal matter moving between the two. Though this happens in less than 1 percent of cases, it requires diverting the intestines into a colostomy bag, so that the fistula can heal without stool moving through the area. Though the colostomy can later be reversed once the complication heals, the experience can be awful. Other rare complications include vaginal stenosis (closing of the vagina if one doesn't dilate properly) and blood clots.

The information was a lot to take in. Meredith and Suzanne learned that because penile and scrotal skin would need to be used to construct part of the vagina if Meredith were to undergo the procedure, she'd need to undergo months of hair removal prior to having the surgery. They decided to start the hair removal process and make consultation appointments with a few surgeons, which couldn't be scheduled for another three months anyway.* They'd continue to reflect on what they learned while they waited for those to be done, before deciding on any next steps.

---

* It's worth noting that some young adult patients in recent years are choosing to have a vulvoplasty only (surgical creation of the external vulva without creation of the vaginal canal) to avoid the need for dilation and hair removal. It is possible to then have a second surgery down the road to create the vaginal canal when the person feels it is a better time to deal with dilation and the more intensive recovery needed for the vaginoplasty.

Meredith continued to meet with Dr. Carey and talk through not only what it would be like to experience surgery, but also what life would be like after either decision (surgery or no surgery). Would she be okay continuing to have a penis? Dr. Carey shared that she cared for many trans women who chose not to have the surgery for all kinds of reasons: being concerned about the risks of surgery, not having genital dysphoria, and some enjoying sex with a penis. Meredith didn't relate to this. While she understood that other trans women might have different experiences, her genital dysphoria made her miserable, and she wanted her genitals to align with her identity. The risks of surgery were scary, and dilation sounded stressful and frustrating, but the decision was still clear in her mind. She explained to Dr. Carey that she didn't share it with other people much because she felt embarrassed, but she'd known since elementary school that she needed to have a vagina.

By the time she got to the initial consultation with her surgeon, her mind was even more firmly made up. And she had spoken with Suzanne about it extensively, who had herself gone through all the medical research in detail, researched the different surgeons around the country who focused on the procedure, and was on board. They drove to New York City and met with a surgeon for the consultation. Because Dr. Carey had worked with patients who had undergone peritoneal vaginoplasties with this surgeon before, Meredith had already known much of the important information, so the consultation didn't have many surprises, though it was nice to hear that the surgeon had a very low complication rate. Meredith and her mom, comfortable with the first consultation, canceled the others and scheduled the surgery for the summer between high school graduation and freshman year.*

Having the surgery scheduled felt like a breath of fresh air for Meredith. She was still nervous, but also excited. She went back to school, going through the motions while waiting for college admissions decisions and her surgery.

On a Wednesday morning, Meredith woke up and went downstairs to the kitchen to make coffee before school. As the coffee dripped through the Keurig and into her Stanford mug (she got it when she went to a summer program there the year before), she took a deep breath in through her nose and slowly out through her mouth as she pursed her lips. It was the day that Stanford early-action admission decisions would come out.

That day, she and her friends didn't talk to each other much. They all sat in class and barely listened to their teachers. She had seen that Stanford decisions would be released at 4:00 p.m. Pacific time, which meant she had to wait until 7:00 p.m. in her time zone. Sitting through classes felt like torture, and she eventually rushed home after school.

She sat on the couch watching the news and told her family she wanted to be alone to try not to think about the decision. At seven, she opened the Stanford online portal and read the letter. She took a deep breath and walked into the kitchen where her parents and brother looked up at her.

---

* Due to the small number of qualified gender-affirming surgeons, the high volume of patients seeking surgery, and subsequent long wait lists, surgeons tell me that it's increasingly rare that they can accommodate this kind of timing request. It tends to be only the most affluent, well-connected families who can arrange for this, creating substantial equity issues.

"I got in!"

The rest of the year was way less academically stressful, and Meredith turned her attention to her upcoming surgery. She graduated from high school and two weeks later was in a hotel in New York City the night before her surgery.

The morning of, she arrived at the hospital at six thirty, accompanied by Suzanne. The surgeon walked in to say hello and did a quick physical exam to make sure the hair removal was successful. After the exam, she looked at Meredith. "Everything looks good—are you ready?"

Meredith said yes, and the surgeon squeezed her hand before letting the anesthesiologist take over.

8

The Science of Gender Politics

Bathrooms, Sports & Legislating Medicine

When I first started working with transgender youth, there were periodic political attacks—you may remember the infamous 2016 battle over North Carolina's HB2—a bill that aimed to force trans people to use the bathrooms that aligned with their sex assigned at birth. But over the past five years or so, political attacks on trans people, and trans kids in particular, have reached a fever pitch. At this time of writing, the American Civil Liberties Union is tracking 501 anti-LGBTQ bills in state legislatures, most of which are aimed at transgender people. The sheer volume of bills targeting my patients has become so large that I can't keep track of them all. And increasingly, the politicians who are working to spread misinformation about these young people are winning—and their laws are passing. In one extreme case, Texan politicians labeled gender affirmation child abuse, leaving families of trans kids in the state horrified that their kids would be taken away from them. Many felt forced to upend their lives and flee to other states.

For people who don't have trans people in their lives, it's easy to overlook what's going on. But if you look closer, you'll quickly realize it's terrifying. And that these are attacks on innocent children and families. My sincerest hope is that this chapter will help you understand the actual science and evidence that should be informing these debates, and that you'll be empowered to spread that information to protect trans youth and their families. I also hope to introduce you to some of the real children who are being negatively impacted, bringing the faces of the victims forward in a space where harm is often discussed on an intellectualized plane.

First and foremost, trans people are being devastated by these political attacks. But at a broader scale, you'll notice that the implications of these antitrans laws go far beyond just trans people. They're both emblematic of, and a driving force for, how public policy and politics are moving away from science and evidence and toward inflammatory emotional rhetoric. They're part of a trend toward politicians attacking others who don't look like them or don't share their personal life experiences. Political actors increasingly don't care if things are true or backed up by evidence, so long as they can get people emotionally riled up and convinced to vote for them. These attacks on transgender people are also related to broader cultural and political changes that involve attacks on due process, the public education system, the LGBTQ community at large, and the ways we approach human rights. Not only do these bills hurt transgender people, but they also hurt our democracy, our approach to legislation, and how we think about human rights and dignity.

THE BATHROOM BATTLEGROUND— WHAT DATA SAY ABOUT TRANS-INCLUSIVE BATHROOM POLICIES

One of the first transgender patients I met at the GeMS clinic in Boston was Nicole Maines. At the time, she was in her early teenage years and had recently started taking estrogen. Her family's story was remarkable. Her dad, Wayne, is an air force veteran, avid outdoorsman, and all-around burly dude. He once described himself as a "solid Ronald Reagan-loving Republican."

He also loves his daughter and struggled for years watching her experience gender dysphoria. By the time I met the Maines family, they had learned to affirm and support her, and Nicole was happy.

But that wasn't always the case. The Maines family struggled with years of harassment related to Nicole's being trans, and it all began with something you've probably heard about before when it comes to trans people: bathrooms.

When Nicole, with her beaming smile, long eyelashes, and shiny brown locks, came out to her elementary school classmates as a girl at age six, her classmates didn't care. Most kids who haven't yet been exposed to transphobia and aren't yet stained by bias don't have the same hang-ups about gender that adults do. Transphobia is not innate, but rather learned as we age.

But in fifth grade, things changed. A new student moved to town and joined Nicole's school. His grandfather, having presumably grown up hearing that transgender people are dangerous and threatening, was alarmed. He was convinced that Nicole using the girls' bathroom was dangerous. Mind you, Nicole had been using it for years by this point, without any issues.

As Nicole explained it, "None of the girls or the girls' families cared." The issue came from this grandfather of a student Nicole barely knew—a male student who didn't even use the girls' bathroom.

That grandfather eventually called the local news and outed Nicole. He was adamant that she posed a danger to the other girls in the bathroom—at nine years old. The grandfather even directed his grandson to go into the girls' bathroom in an attempt to make his point.

Nicole's parents, staunch conservatives who themselves took time to accept their daughter's gender identity, were devastated. They watched Nicole become anxious, depressed, and self-conscious. They were ultimately forced to move to another city.

Forcing trans kids to use bathrooms that don't match their gender identity sends a stigmatizing and painful message to these kids that can negatively impact mental health. But on top of that, such policies also create safety risks.

State legislators introducing "bathroom bills" often say that they are introducing them because they think they will reduce rates of sexual assault. It's an offensive notion that trans people are all sexual assailants. It's also been shown, through objective data, to be false. Cisgender people aren't the ones at risk in public bathrooms—transgender people are.

In 2019, researchers from the Harvard School of Public Health analyzed data from a sample of 3,673 transgender students in grades seven through twelve. Their landmark study, published in the journal *Pediatrics*, found that policies that force transgender youth to use the bathrooms of their sex assigned at birth were associated with dramatically *elevated* rates of sexual assault against transgender kids in schools.

Participants were asked, "During the past twelve months, how many times did anyone force you to do sexual things that you did not want to do? (Count such things as kissing, touching, or being physically forced to have sexual intercourse.)"

The results were shocking: 25.9 percent of participants in the study overall reported that they had been sexually assaulted in the past year alone. Going to a school that forced trans kids to use facilities of their sex assigned at birth was associated with between a 1.3- and 2.5-fold increased risk of sexual assault in the past year. Though researchers didn't ask if the participants had ever been similarly victimized in their full lifetime, those numbers would surely be higher.

Ironically, proponents of bathroom bills to force trans kids to use the bathrooms associated with their sex assigned at birth argue that they are working to *prevent* trauma, when in reality they're generating trauma for kids like Nicole.

While the Harvard study showed that trans-inclusive facility policies are linked to better safety for trans youth, the study didn't look at the impact of such policies for cisgender people or the general population.

However, another study from researchers at UCLA looked at just this. They examined different localities within Massachusetts—some of which had trans-inclusive facility policies—and others that did not. They then submitted public-record requests to analyze the sexual assault rates in each locality. They found that trans-inclusive facility policies were not associated with any increased risk of sexual assault against the general (primarily cisgender) population.

If we look at these two studies together, we see that trans-inclusive public accommodations policies pose no risk to cisgender people, while they are dramatically linked to lower rates of assault against trans young people, in particular. Despite the constant political rhetoric that trans people are dangerous in bathrooms, the reality is that they are *in danger* from people in bathrooms. It's vital that we protect them from being forced into bathrooms and other public facilities that aren't safe for them.

Sadly, these studies rarely make their way into the political rhetoric around bathroom bills that would put young people like Nicole at risk. Transgender people deserve access to public accommodations just like everyone else. Being able to go to school without the risk of being assaulted should be a basic right for students. Trans-inclusive policies create safer, happier communities. This is an area where it is vital that public policy be driven by research and data, rather than political rhetoric that falsely paints trans people as dangerous.

TESTOSTERONE AND ATHLETIC ADVANTAGE—WHY DO POLITICIANS SUDDENLY CARE ABOUT GIRLS' SPORTS?

Over the past two years, one topic has dominated much of the political discussion related to transgender young people: sports participation. The primary question here has been whether transgender girls should be allowed to participate on sports teams that align with their gender identity. Proponents of legislation that would force trans girls to play on boys' sports team argue that trans girls would have an unfair advantage on girls' sports teams. Thus, they argue that trans girls would be taking things like titles and scholarships away from cisgender girls. Many were surprised to see politicians suddenly interested in women's sports, something they never seemed to prioritize in the past. Advocates for women's sports, including the Women's Sports Foundation, had long been raising issues important to them (the lower pay for female athletes, the lesser media coverage for women's sports, cultural environments that lead to high dropout rates for racially and ethnically minoritized athletes)* with very little attention from elected officials. A brief detour into history may explain why politicians have recently focused on this particular type of legislation, and why it's been so successful.

In the late 1980s and early 1990s, cities in Colorado started passing laws prohibiting antigay discrimination. Frustrated

---

* Many of these topics are reviewed in a recent report by the Women's Sports Foundation entitled *Chasing Equity: The Triumphs, Challenges, and Opportunities in Sports for Girls and Women*, published in 2020.

by this social progress, social conservatives in the state created an organization called Colorado for Family Values, and they came up with a bold strategy to stop the state from passing more antidiscrimination laws. They decided to start a ballot initiative to amend the Colorado State constitution to prohibit state and local governments from passing them. They had two public relations strategies. The first was to label LGBTQ people as "groomers" and dangerous to children, a strategy we've seen refurbished in recent years. The second was a more palatable "fairness" argument. They created the false narrative that antidiscrimination laws would give gay people preferential or "better" treatment than straight people. They ran the catchy slogan "Equal rights, not special rights." The strategy was based, in large part, on the fact that the political operatives knew that those working on civil rights issues had hit a snag with affirmative action. Liberal white voters generally supported civil rights, but not when they perceived them as taking something away from them, as they did with affirmative action. It didn't matter that antidiscrimination laws didn't actually take anything away from people. The slogan was catchy; the strategy was successful, and the Colorado constitution was eventually amended.* The same strategy is being recycled today with transgender sports legislation—politicians are painting trans participation in sports as taking something away from cisgender people, in the hopes that this will convince voters to support the bans, and their political movements more broadly.

---

*The U.S. Supreme Court later struck down the amendment as unconstitutional in the 1996 landmark case *Romer v. Evans*.

This brings us to one of the most frequently cited stories of the trans sports debate. In February of 2020, the families of three cisgender girls, supported by the social conservative legal powerhouse the Alliance Defending Freedom,* filed a federal lawsuit against the Connecticut Association of Schools. The families were upset that transgender girls were competing against cisgender girls in school track leagues. They argued that transgender girls have an unfair advantage in high school sports due to their physiology and should therefore be forced to play on boys' teams.

One columnist summed up the Alliance Defending Freedom argument about the Connecticut case in the *Wall Street Journal*: when transgender girls compete on girls' sports teams, "[cisgender] girls can't win."

The writer of course left out the fact that one of the cisgender girls from that lawsuit beat the transgender girls named in the lawsuit in the Connecticut state track championship just two days after the case was filed.

I reached out to Andraya Yearwood, one of the transgender girls who was brought into the case. She joined me on Zoom from her parents' house, on summer break from college at North Carolina Central University. She had just finished her sophomore year and was getting ready to study abroad in Argentina for her junior year.

---

* The Alliance Defending Freedom is the same group that was behind the recent Supreme Court case *Dobbs v. Jackson Women's Health Organization* (2022), which overturned *Roe v. Wade*. They also argued for the criminalization of homosexuality in amicus briefs for the U.S. Supreme Court Case *Lawrence v. Texas* (2003). However, in *Lawrence*, the Court ultimately ruled that so-called sodomy laws were unconstitutional.

Despite the difficult experiences she had around the court case, Andraya had a bright, happy demeanor. Her smile was nonstop throughout our chat, and she frequently flipped her long braids over her shoulder when she spoke. Her voice and demeanor revealed a confidence and comfort with herself that's rare for people her age.

She explained to me that she came out as transgender in middle school and at that time continued to compete on the boys' team. But when she made it to high school, the administrators there told her that if she was going to live as a girl in every other aspect of life, she should run on the girls' track team, too.

Andraya's parents are warm and caring and have always supported her gender expression. I suspect this is why she has the comfortable demeanor she has. When she joined the high school girls' track team, her coach and teammates were just as embracing.

Andraya admits that she didn't see the controversy coming. She and her friend Terry, who is also a trans girl, had been running on the team without any issues. While we spoke, Andraya scrolled through her Instagram messages and found some direct messages from one of the cisgender girls who was a plaintiff from the lawsuit. All the messages back and forth were of them congratulating each other for doing well at meets.

Andraya heard about the lawsuit the day before the Connecticut state track championships. She remembers feeling shaken. Not only did she need to worry about her performance at the meet, but she also had to worry about a storm of media attention. When she arrived at the track, a security guard was there and followed her around. At one point, she turned and asked him to step back, but he told her he couldn't because he needed to protect her. She felt her feet pull down to the earth as the situation became real.

When it came to her big race, Andraya false started and was disqualified. To this day, she's not sure what happened. "Maybe I was just so in my head and distracted from the chaos. . . . I don't know." She stayed at the meet to watch Terry run. Terry ended up losing to one of the cisgender girls named in the lawsuit. She walked off the track crying, and Andraya followed to console her.

During the media frenzy, attacks against Andraya were vicious. Somehow it was lost on people that the target of their vitriol was a high school student. She remembers seeing people post pictures of her on Twitter, circling the muscle definition on her arms and legs to justify why she shouldn't be running. The attacks were degrading and dehumanizing.

They also seemed to be tinged with racism in addition to transphobia. It was hard to overlook the fact that the two transgender high school students making national news on this issue were both African American and that the cisgender girls from the lawsuit, who were regularly praised on conservative media platforms, were white. It harkened back to a past when people argued that African American athletes needed to be segregated in sports because of a presumed "biological advantage."

Ultimately, the court case about Andraya was thrown out by a federal judge. Because one of the cisgender girls named in the lawsuit beat Andraya and Terry at the state championship, it seemed clear that the argument centered on their being unbeatable wasn't going to hold up. The decision was appealed to the U.S. Court of Appeals for the Second Circuit, which reaffirmed the district court decision, while also noting that discrimination against transgender students violates Title IX, which prohibits sex-based discrimination in schools and other educational programs that receive funding from the federal government.[*]

Despite several victories in court, the case had a lasting impact on Andraya and Terry. In contrast to all the talk in the news about transgender girls "stealing" athletic scholarships from cisgender girls, neither Andraya nor Terry run track in college, and neither received track scholarships. Andraya is lucky to have supportive friends and a loving family who shielded her mental health from being too impacted by the experience. But it nonetheless did turn track, once a fun experience and an important emotional outlet, into something painful. Instead of track, Andraya was focusing on her studies and planned to improve her Spanish skills during her study abroad time in Argentina, while volunteering for some of the major feminist organizations in South America.

In the years to come, politicians in more than twenty U.S. states introduced legislation that would force transgender girls to play on boys' sports teams.

Many, including me, saw this as a political attack on trans people that wasn't based on an actual problem. Were trans athletes dominating sports leagues? To look into this question, journalists at the Associated Press reached out to two dozen state legislators who'd introduced such legislation and asked if

---

[*] In December 2023, the U.S. Court of Appeals for the Second Circuit revived the case for ongoing consideration.

they could name a transgender athlete in their state. The vast majority couldn't name a single one, let alone cite any evidence suggesting that trans people were dominating sports leagues or were overrepresented among sports title holders.

Utah became one of the states in which legislators voted for a law that would force trans youth to play on sports teams that aligned with their sex assigned at birth. In response, Republican governor Spencer Cox vetoed the legislation. In a public statement explaining his veto, he pointed out that there were only four transgender students competing in the state and that only one of those was playing on a girls' team. His statement went on to say, "Four kids who are just trying to find some friends and feel like they are part of something. Four kids trying to get through each day . . . rarely has so much fear and anger been directed at so few."

State lawmakers largely ignored his remarks and voted to override his veto, making Utah the twelfth state to implement a ban targeting transgender athletes. Families of trans youth in Utah subsequently filed a lawsuit to block enforcement of the law. A similar lawsuit was filed after Idaho passed its trans sports bill, and the federal courts blocked enforcement of the law pending the ongoing court case.*

There's plenty of reason to think that trans youth don't pose a risk to women's sports. California passed a law in 2013 protecting the rights of transgender students to play on teams that match their gender identity. There have been no issues. Similarly, the Olympics have allowed transgender athletes to

---

* For disclosure, I filed an expert-witness statement in this Idaho case on behalf of those suing the state to block the law from going into effect.

compete in the categories that align with their gender identities since 2004. Despite this policy, not a single openly transgender athlete qualified for the Olympics until the 2021 games. Most notable among those who qualified was weight lifter Laurel Hubbard, a transgender woman who was attacked by the media for having an "unfair advantage," yet was eliminated after just three lifts. The only transgender Olympic athlete to win a medal that year was the mononymous Quinn, a nonbinary Canadian women's soccer player whose team won gold. Quinn was assigned female at birth, so the team's victory can't be used as evidence that people assigned male at birth are taking over women's sports.

The idea that transgender girls will dominate girls' sports is based on the presumption that transgender girls are exposed to higher levels of testosterone during puberty, and that this exposure causes physical changes—including an increase in muscle mass—that cisgender girls don't experience. However, an estimated 10 percent of cisgender girls have polycystic ovary syndrome, which leads to elevated testosterone. No politicians have proposed banning them from sports or forcing them to participate on boys' teams. Transgender girls who take puberty blockers, on the other hand, have negligible testosterone levels, yet these proposed laws would force them to compete on boys' sports teams. To complicate things further, the athletic advantage conferred by testosterone is constantly debated. As Dr. Katrina Karkazis, senior visiting fellow at Yale and expert on testosterone and bioethics, explained to me, "Studies of testosterone levels in athletes do not show any clear consistent relationship between testosterone and athletic performance. Sometimes testosterone is associated with better performance, but other times studies show weak or no links."

Some politicians point to studies showing that cisgender men outperform cisgender women in certain competitions. Though political pundits may try to say that transgender women are just cisgender men, it's vital to remember that this isn't true.

In a 2023 commentary in the peer-reviewed journal *Sports Medicine*, three experts reviewed the many reasons this assumption doesn't hold up. For example, they pointed to a study showing that transgender women have 6.8 percent less lean mass than cisgender men, even before starting any kind of gender-affirming hormones.

Transgender girls also suffer from dramatically higher rates of bullying, harassment, anxiety, and depression when compared to cisgender girls. All these things make it harder to train and succeed in sports, and they are likely reasons why transgender people are underrepresented both in sports participation and titles. A 2017 survey of over seventeen thousand youth found that while 68 percent of the national sample of youth played on a sports team, only 12 percent of the transgender girls in the study reported participating on a team. The reality is that, when it comes to sports, transgender youth are at a profound *disadvantage* and are underrepresented.

Perhaps if we make it to a future in which transphobia and harassment of trans people recede, some sort of testosterone advantage will be revealed, and we'll start to see more trans women dominating sports leagues. But this is theoretical, and today's reality is that trans people are disadvantaged in nearly every way in our society, including in sports. In talking about these bills, we need to also consider the mental health impact they have on people. Forcing a transgender girl to play on a boys' sports team is cruel and invalidating.

Living in an accepting part of New England, Meredith has been lucky that she's always been allowed to participate in girls' activities at school. She spent years playing on the field hockey team. "I just wanted to hang out with my friends. I couldn't imagine being told I could live as myself throughout the day, but once school ends, be told I'm a boy and need to go play on the boys' team."

Realistically, most transgender children will not play sports if they are banned from teams that match their gender identity. They will therefore miss out on the important benefits that team sports and physical activity can have for their mental and physical health.

This is particularly relevant when it comes to bone health. We talked earlier about how important it is to monitor bone density when pursuing gender-affirming medical care, given that adolescents tend to fall behind on bone density when on pubertal suppression. It turns out that trans youth have lower bone density than cisgender youth even prior to starting any gender-affirming medical interventions. This is often attributed to the fact that trans youth get less physical activity compared to cisgender youth, likely in part due to the stigma trans youth face when playing school sports. In an editorial in the journal *Pediatrics*, Drs. Laura Bachrach and Catherine Gordon noted, "Young transgender youth may worry about teasing by peers while engaging in sports, thereby discouraging them from these activities in a school or community setting." Now that this teasing is not just from peers but also from powerful politicians, it would not be surprising if we see even fewer trans youth participating in sports, and subsequently facing physical health consequences.

Team sports have also been shown to have important social and emotional benefits for young people. In 2022, a team of researchers published a study in the journal *PLoS One* based on data from over eleven thousand youth ages nine to thirteen. They found that, when compared to kids who didn't participate in team sports, those who participated had lower rates of a range of mental health problems including depression and anxiety. For young trans people who already suffer from dramatically elevated rates of anxiety and depression, team sports can give them a sense of social connection, acceptance, and validation that can make a huge positive impact. But this can only happen if the teams are safe and supportive.

For many kids, sports are also a coping mechanism—a way for them to deal with feelings of anxiety or depression. When Kentucky introduced a bill to ban trans youth from playing on sports teams that align with their gender identity, seventh grader Fischer Wells testified in front of lawmakers, "I really don't want this bill to pass because that means I can't play, and it will be extremely detrimental to my mental health as well, because I know that sports is a great way for me to cope with things." Fischer was the only known transgender athlete in the state and had helped to start her school's girls' field hockey team in Louisville.

Even for the kids who are too afraid to play sports, the conversations we're having around sports participation are impacting them. When I talked to Kyle about recent bills that aim to kick trans kids off sports teams that match their gender identity, he shared with me, "Listen, I don't care about sports, but it's hard to read in the media every day about people who think people like me aren't valid. It's hard not to take those messages to heart. Why does everyone hate me? Maybe there is something wrong with me."

Kyle's comments reminded me of an important topic we often think about when it comes to the mental health of LGBTQ youth—the minority stress theory. The theory was first popularized by UCLA psychiatric epidemiologist Ilan Meyer in 1995 (at the time, he was a professor at Columbia University in New York City). Dr. Meyer described something that was novel then but may seem obvious to most of us today—that the way society treats minoritized people impacts their mental health.

When he first described minority stress, he applied it primarily to gay men. Later in 2012, psychologists noted that a similar phenomenon applied to transgender people, which we often refer to as the gender minority stress framework.

The first part of the theory is intuitive—that so-called distal stressors (I think of them as external factors—things outside us), like harassment and discrimination, can lead people to feel more depressed and anxious.

The second set of stressors are somewhat less obvious: proximal stressors (I think of them as internal factors—things inside our own minds). The minority stress framework explains that as people are exposed to constant negative messages about trans people, they eventually start to internalize those ideas. We refer to this as internalized transphobia.

It's something I sadly see commonly among my patients. I once sat with a seventeen-year-old transgender boy who told me, "I know that there's nothing wrong with being trans, but it's hard to shake these messages I constantly hear on TV. It's like they're sinking into my brain. Every once in a while, my brain will say, 'Maybe you are a risk to people in bathrooms' or 'Maybe you are dangerous to your soccer friends' or 'Maybe you are just mentally ill and broken—maybe you need to be fixed.' I know these things are absurd, but they still nag at me."

It's not hard to imagine how this would lead to problems with self-esteem and to anxiety and depression over time. Some have pointed out that the constant stress can also lead to other physical problems such as heart disease, as stress hormones constantly flood the system.

The gender minority stress framework describes another proximal stress factor, called negative expectations. You can imagine that if you spend much of your life being a victim of harassment and discrimination, you will expect this in the future, even if you move into a new more affirming environment. It's similar to what psychiatrists see in post-traumatic stress disorder. Let's say I have a patient who was in an awful car accident and needed surgery. That person may become convinced that by getting in another car it will happen again, even though that's extremely unlikely. When people experience a trauma, they tend to overestimate how likely the trauma is to happen again. The same thing happens with minority stress.

I've experienced it myself. Throughout much of my childhood, I was afraid that if anyone found out I was gay, something awful would happen. I thought I'd be beat up by kids at school or disowned by my dad. I was horrified of *anyone* finding out, so I always worked to make sure I hid any sign of being gay. I walked with my stiff posture and deepened my voice. Always.

Now that I live in San Francisco, there's honestly a very low likelihood that I'll be harassed based on my sexual orientation. And yet when I meet someone new or go into a store, I get anxious. I'll deepen my voice and be afraid people will think less of me for being gay, even if I don't really have much reason to think that's going to happen. This is the proximal factor "negative expectations."

My attempts to deepen my voice and walk without any hint of gayness relate to a third major proximal factor: concealment. People over time learn to hide their sexual or gender minority identity, which leads to shame and secrecy, which also worsen anxiety and depression.

The good news from the minority stress framework is that it describes some "resilience factors"—ways in which people can buffer against the negative impacts distal and proximal stressors tend to have on mental health. The first is community connectedness—meeting and forging relationships with other queer people.

A great example of this is TrevorSpace, an online forum created by the Trevor Project, a suicide prevention organization that also provides a mental health crisis hotline for sexual and gender minority young people. TrevorSpace is moderated by adults to keep it appropriate and safe and allows young trans kids to network and meet other kids like them. It lets them learn that they're not alone and helps fight the notion that they're invalid or "uniquely broken"—distorted thoughts that can commonly sneak in as a result of minority stress.

The second major resilience factor is pride. It's important for young trans people to know that trans people have made major contributions in just about every area of society.

In my office, I've hung photos of several trans trailblazers: Rachel Levine (assistant U.S. secretary of health, who founded Penn State's division of adolescent medicine), Chase Strangio (ACLU lawyer who won major Supreme Court cases including marriage equality), Lana and Lilly Wachowski (creators of *The Matrix* and *V for Vendetta*), Martine Rothblatt (creator of Sirius Satellite Radio and the highest-paid female CEO in 2013), Laverne Cox (Emmy Award–winning actress), Quinn (Olympic gold medalist), and many more. It's important that trans youth be able to see role models who look like them.

While debates around sports participation for trans people have been framed as being just about testosterone and athletic advantage, they're really about so much more. They're about human dignity and respect. They're about letting kids be who they are. And they've very much about mental health. At the end of the day—do we really want people to be defined by their genitals, or do we want to see them as whole people?

FROM SHOCK THERAPY TO HORSE FARMS— THE INSIDIOUS HISTORY OF CONVERSION "THERAPY" AND LEGISLATION BANNING THE PRACTICE

Every major medical and mental health organization has labeled attempts to force transgender people to be cisgender dangerous and unethical, given that they are linked to suicide attempts. These efforts are colloquially called transgender conversion therapies, though in the academic literature, we call them gender identity conversion efforts, to highlight that they are not therapeutic. Roughly half of U.S. states have made it illegal to conduct gender identity conversion efforts on minors. However, there has been a persistent movement among political actors to try to get the courts to overturn the laws. There's reason to worry that they may be successful. Before jumping into the politics and law, it's essential to hear the actual human experience of conversion therapy.

The story of Carolyn Mercer highlights just how devastating these practices can be. On a dull autumn day in 1964, in a hospital in Lancashire, England, seventeen-year-old Carolyn was strapped to a wooden chair in a dark room, with electrodes attached to her arm. Doctors projected pictures of women's clothing on the screen in front of her and sent painful electric shocks into her arm with each picture. Though tears of agony rolled down her face during the sessions, the doctors continued the treatment for months. They hoped that if Carolyn associated femininity with pain, she would be "cured" of being transgender and come to identify as male.

They were wrong. Carolyn developed PTSD and started to have flashbacks and uncontrolled shaking anytime something reminded her of the shock therapy. In addition to her PTSD symptoms, Carolyn explained that the treatment made her hate herself more than she already did, throwing her into a deep depression. Now seventy-four years old, she is more comfortable living as herself, but her treatment caused her irreparable psychological harm. As she told the BBC, "I don't have a light anymore, or emotion like that, because I suppressed it for so long."

When they think of conversion therapy, most people think of attempts to force gay people to be straight. This is called sexual orientation conversion therapy. Gender identity conversion therapy is different.* It refers to attempts to force transgender people to be cisgender. Over the years it has taken many forms, from shock therapy such as Carolyn's to less physically painful but still psychologically scarring approaches. In 2019, our research group published a study estimating that hundreds of thousands of transgender people in the United States have been exposed to the practice.

The ways in which conversion efforts are practiced have evolved substantially. Nowadays, we rarely hear about aversive shock therapy approaches such as those Carolyn experienced. But even in the recent academic literature, you can find examples of gender identity conversion effort approaches. As mentioned in the parent-blaming chapter, in 2002, Columbia University psychologist Heino Meyer-Bahlburg published a paper in the journal *Clinical Child Psychology and Psychiatry* entitled "Gender Identity Disorder in Young Boys: A Parent- and Peer-Based Treatment Protocol."† Though the protocol did not describe itself as a conversion effort manual, it did contain a section entitled "Justification of Treatment," in which it noted the goal of treatment was to "speed up the fading of the cross-gender identity." The protocol itself included such things as taking the child out of playdates with girls, putting them in male-typical activities such as Scouts,

---

* Though the definitions are different, legal scholar and bioethicist Florence Ashley has pointed out in her 2022 book, *Banning Transgender Conversion Practices*, that the practices share some similarities in how they are operationalized.

† It's worth noting that the approach was meant to be used only for prepubertal children, as the consensus in the field, even then, was that trans identities were largely stable and unmodifiable after puberty began.

and "letting go of the boy by the mother." While it didn't recommend any aversive techniques like punishment for gender diverse behavior, it's hard to imagine that children didn't experience shame as their parents pushed them into gender roles with which they didn't identify. The manual also included a list of "putative gender risk factors," including sexual abuse, sibling rivalry, feminine physical appearance, and maternal dominance, which, as discussed earlier, have no real empiric basis.

In some cases, parents seem to attempt conversion efforts without working with a therapist. In the book *Irreversible Damage*, the author interviews a family that believed their child came to be transgender as a result of social media influences. According to the author, the family sent their child to a horse farm with no internet or phone access, hoping that the isolation would cause the child to become cisgender. The author of the book asserts that children whose parents isolated them in this way all "desisted" from being transgender. It is, of course, also possible, and in my opinion much more likely, that these children were traumatized by the experience and went back in the closet to avoid being subjected to future conversion efforts.

The "Justification of Treatment" section of Meyer-Bahlburg's paper goes on to say that he hoped to make these children cisgender to avoid the harassment from peers that such kids often face, as well as to prevent the need for gender-affirming medical interventions in the future, which of course carry side effects.

These concerns are ones that I often hear from the parents of transgender youth, and both are very real concerns. It's important for clinicians to validate the worries parents have, as they represent a healthy desire to protect their children. However, families and their care teams also must weigh the considerable risks of the conversion efforts against these other risks. They should also work with schools and communities to change their bullying behaviors, rather than trying to change the child.

In 2019, our research group published a study in the journal *JAMA Psychiatry* examining associations between exposure to gender identity conversion efforts and mental health outcomes. The study included a sample of over twenty-seven thousand transgender adults from all fifty U.S. states and territories abroad. We found that, when compared to people who had therapy without gender identity conversion efforts, those who were exposed to conversion efforts had more than double the odds of having attempted suicide in their lifetime. If they were exposed to conversion efforts as prepubertal children (the target population in Meyer-Bahlburg's paper), the association with suicidality was even more dramatic—a fourfold increased odds of attempting suicide.* We found that it didn't matter whether these conversion efforts came from secular professionals like therapists or from religious advisers—the associations with suicidality were the same.

Some people get confused about the difference between "gender exploratory psychotherapy" and conversion efforts. With exploratory psychotherapy, people meet with a therapist with the goal of better understanding their gender. The important thing here is that exploratory psychotherapy is open-ended, nondirective, and has no predetermined gender identity goal. Conversion efforts, in contrast, have the explicit

---

* This was after adjusting for potential other variables that could impact the results, including family support of gender identity and socioeconomic status.

goal of a person's becoming cisgender as a result of therapy. Sadly, some people appear to be practicing conversion efforts under the false label of *exploratory psychotherapy*, presumably in an attempt to shield themselves from repercussions, since all major medical organizations, including the American Psychiatric Association and the American Academy of Child & Adolescent Psychiatry have labeled gender identity conversion efforts dangerous and unethical.

Though the topic is understudied, it appears that most such therapists practice in states in which conversion efforts are still legal. Twenty states and Washington, DC, have passed bans on the practice; however, this means that it is still legal in most U.S. states.

To complicate policy matters further, antitrans legal organizations have brought legal challenges regarding the constitutionality of conversion effort bans. In three such cases, in the U.S. Courts of Appeals for the Third and Ninth Circuits, judges have ruled that such bans are in fact constitutional, upholding them.

But in 2020, the U.S. Court of Appeals for the Eleventh Circuit, led by Trump-appointed judges, ruled that two conversion effort bans in Florida were unconstitutional. Their decision included an argument that such bans were an infringement upon the free speech rights of therapists who practice conversion efforts.* They went on to acknowledge that

---

* For those interested in the legal complexities, the other courts ruled that speech that is "incidental to conduct" such as practicing medicine is generally not protected in this way and can be limited when a state has a compelling interest in maintaining public safety.

the American Psychiatric Association has labeled conversion efforts dangerous and unethical; however, they then asserted that the organization cannot be trusted because it once labeled homosexuality a disease and no longer does. These convoluted attacks on scientific progress and human rights are alarming. The notion that professional organizations cannot make progress in their understanding of best practices is a slippery slope that allows courts to essentially discount all scientific evidence.

This is a problem not constrained to conversion effort bans. Justice Amy Coney Barrett insisted during her Supreme Court confirmation hearing that climate change is not established science, and there is concern that she will similarly argue that the harms of conversion efforts are not established, despite substantial evidence and the broad consensus among the medical and scientific communities.

Given that federal circuit courts now have divergent opinions regarding the constitutionality of conversion effort bans, it is likely that the question will go to the Supreme Court. With the court's current composition and recent rhetoric, there is strong reason to believe the court will rule to overturn conversion efforts bans throughout the United States, putting countless young people at risk.

POLITICIANS IN THE PEDIATRICIAN'S OFFICE— GOVERNMENT ATTEMPTS TO LIMIT ACCESS TO GENDER-AFFIRMING CARE FOR TRANSGENDER YOUTH

Despite gender-affirming medical care for adolescents with gender dysphoria being endorsed by all major medical organizations, several states have attempted to pass legislation to make the practice illegal.

In February of 2020, the South Dakota House of Representatives passed a bill called HB1057: the Vulnerable Child Protection Act. The bill would have made gender-affirming medical treatments for adolescent gender dysphoria illegal, punishable with jail time. I was surprised to see it pass even one chamber of the state's legislature. I admit that at the time I didn't take the bill—introduced by a relatively unknown chiropractor-politician, Fred Deutsch—very seriously. I wrote a piece about the proposed law for the *New York Times*, explaining why it was a bad idea, and when the bill failed to pass the South Dakota Senate, I assumed that was the end of it. I could not have been more wrong.

As of September 2023, the Human Rights Campaign reported that twenty-two states had passed laws or policies banning gender-affirming medical care for trans youth, with several other states considering similar laws in their legislative bodies. Most had been challenged in court, and the challenges were often successful.* Even Trump-appointed federal judges in Alabama and Indiana issued preliminary injunctions against the laws, blocking their enforcement until a full trial could be held. In his opinion, Trump-appointed Alabama judge Liles Burke wrote, "Parent plaintiffs have a fundamental right to direct the medical care of their children" and "at least twenty-two major medical associations in the United States endorse transitioning medications [*sic*] as well-established, evidence-based treatment for gender

---

* For disclosure, I have served as an expert witness in several of these cases.

dysphoria in minors." At the time of writing, the only ban on gender-affirming medical care for transgender youth that has gone through a full trial is in Arkansas, where a federal judge ruled the law was unconstitutional. The state subsequently appealed to the Eighth Circuit.

Despite this, the sheer volume of introduced bills creates concern that many of them will ultimately go into effect, taking this medical care away from adolescents who need it.* Republicans appear to have made bans on gender-affirming medical care a major priority, and they have developed highly effective rhetoric around it. Political pundits on outlets such as Fox News are often heard using terms such as "genital mutilation" and "experimentation on children" to scare voters into supporting medical care bans. As we've talked about here, none of this rhetoric is accurate. Gender-affirming genital surgery is rarely performed on minors, and never on young children. Gender-affirming medical care also isn't experimental—over a dozen studies have linked treatments such as pubertal suppression and gender-affirming hormones to better mental health outcomes for adolescents. Among them is a recent study of 315 adolescents with gender dysphoria, published in the prestigious *New England Journal of Medicine*, which found improvements

---

* As I edit this again in November of 2023, there has been rapid movement in the courts on this topic. U.S. Circuit Courts of Appeals for the Eleventh and Sixth Circuits have overturned preliminary injunctions that had put enforcement of some of these bills on hold while full trials proceeded. The ACLU, which opposes bans on gender-affirming medical care for adolescent gender dysphoria, has appealed one of those decisions to the U.S. Supreme Court. Of note, both appellate decisions allowing bans to go into effect cited the recent Supreme Court case *Dobbs v. Jackson Women's Health* (which overturned *Roe v. Wade*).

in anxiety, depression, and life satisfaction after treatment. But the average person isn't well-versed in the nuances of gender-affirming care, nor the research on it, resulting in these bans garnering substantial support among the electorate. Most aren't aware that every relevant major medical organization has explicitly opposed bans on gender-affirming medical care for adolescent gender dysphoria, including the American Medical Association, the American Psychiatric Association, the American Academy of Pediatrics, and the American Academy of Child & Adolescent Psychiatry, among others.

Attacks on gender-affirming medical care for adolescent gender dysphoria aren't limited to the United States. In the United Kingdom, a high court ordered that minors could not consent to puberty blockers without a judge first ruling that they understand the treatment. This ruling was confusing for those practicing medicine in the United States, since outside of very specific circumstances, it is assumed that minors lack the ability to consent for medications on their own, meaning parents need to provide the consent. A later case in the United Kingdom emphasized this point, and a higher court there also ultimately overturned the initial ruling that had limited youth's access to pubertal suppression. The United Kingdom similarly saw misinformation permeate their courts, with that initial decision falsely claiming that puberty blockers make kids more likely to "persist" in their transgender identity.

Parents of transgender youth are horrified by this legislation. In one qualitative study of 273 parents of trans youth, they overwhelmingly expressed fear that such legislation would lead to worsening mental health and increased suicidal ideation for their children, with one parent stating, "This could mean death for my child."

The laws (and related executive actions) have even caused some families to flee their states. Soon after politicians in Texas circumvented the state legislature to label gender-affirming medical care "child abuse" and directed their child protective services to investigate parents who affirm their transgender children, I met with the Shappley family.

Kimberly Shappley was wearing thick-rimmed black glasses, with her hair carefully tucked behind her ears. Sharp bangs cut across her forehead, and big cheeks amplified her eyes, which were tinged with sadness, fear, and anger through-out different parts of our meeting. Her eleven-year-old daugh-ter, Kai, was sitting next to her, wearing a flowing yellow blouse and blushing at the prospect of talking to a stranger, but also clearly excited. Despite the family's awful experiences with the political environment in Texas, Kai was bubbly. She sat self-assured, with her blond hair in pigtails.

Kai introduced herself to me and told me her pronouns were "*her/she*—like the chocolate bar." Kim told me her pro-nouns were the same, then told me their family's story. Kai had started telling her mom at age three and a half that she was a girl. Kim, a conservative Christian, was told by her church that she needed to punish Kai each time she said this. These punishments would range from spankings to time-outs, and each time with a reminder to Kai that she "was a boy." Despite this, Kai continued to insist that she was a girl. Kim finally had a breaking point when she heard Kai praying to "be with Jesus forever so she could be a girl with him." It was a slow process, but Kim realized she needed to do something different, so she let Kai socially transition by growing out her hair and using new pronouns and a new name. The change wasn't accepted by their small town in Texas, which led them to move to Austin, hoping they could live life more peacefully.

The directive from Texas governor Greg Abbott for child protective services to investigate families didn't come as a complete surprise to Kim when it was issued. Abbott had indicated that if the bill that was introduced in the state legislature to ban gender-affirming care didn't pass, that he would still make it so through an executive action. Despite this, news that the directive was official took Kim's breath away. She recounted sitting on the couch crying and shaking while thinking, "I can't keep doing this—it's been six years of trauma on top of trauma on top of trauma . . . just when you first start healing, you get retraumatized." By this point, Kim's family had already stopped talking to her because of Kai's being trans. She had needed to change jobs to get insurance that would cover the puberty blocker Kai started when she was eight. She had been asked to step away from the boards of churches she sat on and had lost much of the Christian religious community that was so important to her. But Kai had become a completely different child once she was affirmed—vibrant and self-assured. Kim would do anything to make sure her child stayed that way.

Kim was a nurse and told me at the time that she couldn't afford to move out of Texas but was considering it. Several months later when I checked in with her again, the family had sold their house and moved to a safer state,* worried that if they stayed in Texas, Kai might be taken away. Though the burden of

---

* Kim asked me not to name the new state to protect their privacy.

leaving everything behind and moving to a new state was awful, Kim told me it was a huge relief to finally feel safe.

Kai, resilient as ever, was also sad to have needed to upend their life (and leave behind their chickens), but she remains a fierce advocate for herself. When I asked her what she wanted to tell other trans kids going through similar things, she firmly told me, "Just be yourself. Stay strong and stay fabulous."

9

An Eye on the Future

How Gender and Society
Will Continue to Evolve

Over the past several years, more and more physicians and scientists have made their way onto X (formerly Twitter) to build community and educate the public. I've been there for years trying, to the best of my ability, to correct the misinformation that goes around regarding trans youth, and in particular their mental health and medical care. I also try to highlight trans success and joy, to combat what sometimes feels like constant negative messaging about trans young people.

One morning, I decided to make a collage of photos of successful trans people in America to post and remind people that the trans community is beautiful and thriving. Despite how hard things are right now with political attacks on trans people—and trans youth in particular—we've made some amazing strides. The collage highlighted the same trans trailblazers I've hung in my office for patients to see. It showed inspiring leaders in just about every area of American life: medicine (Rachel Levine), law (Chase Strangio), business (Martine Rothblatt), the arts (the Wachowski sisters), sports (Chris Mosier), acting and tech (Angelica Ross), you name it.

One of the trans heroes in the collage was Nicole Maines, the young girl I wrote about earlier in the book, who faced harassment around using her school's bathroom in Maine. Nicole is now twenty-five, and I recently caught up with her on Zoom in between her many acting gigs. After the harassment she faced as a child, Nicole eventually finished high school and went to the University of Maine alongside her twin brother. During college, she started to pursue acting, and her career quickly took off. In 2015, she landed a role in the USA Network show *Royal Pains*. A few years later, she starred as Nia Nal on the CW series *Supergirl*, becoming the first literal trans super-hero on television. When I met with her that afternoon, she had just finished up some filming for the popular Showtime series *Yellowjackets*.

Nicole was sitting at the desk in her apartment, her brown hair with blond highlights cascading down her shoulders. She wore stylish blue glasses that magnified her cheekbones. She looked like a TV star who was having a casual day at home. A still of the Zoom would have looked like a typical casual-glamorous *TMZ* paparazzo photo.

I asked her what was new since I saw her last (I first met Nicole when she was a patient at Boston Children's Hospital back in the early 2010s).* She was quick to tell me that gender-affirming care gave her the opportunity to be the best version of herself, "the most ambitious and creative person [she] could be." She described a huge transformation in her life once she finally saw a way forward with her transition. "Once I was finally given a clear path, I was able to focus on this best version of myself, and I thrived. I'm a comic book writer, an award-winning actress, and I just did season two of *Yellowjackets*, the most popular show on television. I wouldn't have been able to do all this if I were still consumed with being stuck feeling like a prisoner in my own body."

She explained that she hardly ever thinks about the fact that she's trans. "It's not like I wake up in the morning and say I'm going to go make some trans toast and get ready for my trans day spreading the trans agenda. I super don't care." Her focus was on her career, enjoying her new group of friends since she had moved to Los Angeles, and her new partner, Nate. She let me know that Nate is supportive. "He just doesn't give a fuck. He doesn't care about the trans thing. He just sees me as his girlfriend, and that's enough for him." She explained that people get so heated, building transness up to be a huge thing in their head, and it doesn't need to be. Half-journalist, half-nosy, I did later google Nate and found some media coverage of their relationship. A *Pride* story about them quoted Nate as referring to Nicole as "a peak in my life."

I asked Nicole how she felt about where things are in America today and asked her where she thinks things are going. The

---

* Nicole has given me permission to talk about this and has been public about her experiences at GeMS.

tone of her voice became more serious. But she said as dreadful as things are now, she thinks it's this way because we have made so much progress for trans people, and people who don't understand or know trans people are freaking out in response. She told me it sometimes feels as if trans people are screaming from the rooftops about how scary the backlash has been, and that there is no one there to protect them. She hopes that everyone will chip in so that we can combat antitrans sentiments, and she explained that everyone has a stake, since it seems unlikely that the politicians attacking trans people are going to stop at just trans groups if they succeed—she suspects other minority groups will be next. Her comment reminded me of a 2022 concurring opinion penned by Supreme Court justice Clarence Thomas for *Dobbs v. Jackson Women's Health Organization*, in which he signaled his interest in overturning past judicial decisions that protected gay marriage and access to contraception. Often, attacking one marginalized group serves as an entryway to attack others, taking baby steps toward normalizing such attacks, until people feel accustomed to them.

On a hopeful note, Nicole thinks people *are* starting to catch on to what's happening: history is repeating its attack on a marginalized group just as what happened in America with people of color, gay people, and women. She's holding out hope that people will see through the rhetoric, and we'll make progress the way we have in other areas of human rights. She posed this question to people still considering "both sides" of transgender public policies: "What do you think is more likely: that there's an entire group of people who are groomers and pedophiles all engaging in a multi-million-dollar conspiracy to trans your children, or do you think maybe the same politicians who have perpetrated violence and discrimination against every other marginalized group throughout history are maybe still doing that?"

While Nicole and I had tackled some tough topics, I left our meeting with a strong sense of hope. Nicole was amazing. She was confident, eloquent, charismatic, and thriving both professionally and personally. We are in a time in which people like Nicole who received gender-affirming care from early in life can be on television and be role models. She had just finished filming a segment for PBS on trans rights that will be coming out soon. The stereotype of what trans people are was being updated and challenged, and the general public is going to start seeing more people like Nicole. As she wrapped up telling me about the new graphic novel she's writing (an origin story for the superhero Dreamer) and we were saying goodbye, she looked at me with a big smile and said, "I'm glad to see you're doing well." I took a pause. We spend so much time worrying about trans youth and all that they're up against in today's society that we often forget that, when people are loved, supported, and affirmed as Nicole was, they thrive. And that there are countless trans young adults out there who are thriving the way she is. It didn't seem to even cross Nicole's mind that I would be worried about her. She didn't need my concern; she was concerned about *me*. How beautiful will a future be where that's the typical trans experience?

MEREDITH

I caught up with Meredith again in August of 2022, about a year after her surgery. She logged into the Zoom room we were meeting in and was framed by a beanbag on one side and an IKEA armoire on the other. She had the same bright smile I remembered from when she was younger, and her curly hair still draped down to her shoulders. Her perfect posture hadn't changed either, and she spoke with a marked confidence and calm. She let me know she was in her new dorm room, having recently returned to Stanford for her sophomore year. She had just finished up a Spanish immersion program in South America, living with a host family. It was a rewarding experience, but one of the first times in her life that, for safety reasons, she told me she needed to go "stealth" and not tell anyone she was trans. It had pushed her to reflect more on how difficult it is for most people to be trans in this world. She was left feeling grateful for the life she was born into, which allowed her to be openly herself. After the study-abroad trip, she spent a few weeks traveling around Europe with her boyfriend, who was a much-needed support system for her to recover and feel more settled in combating the "gaslighting shame" that had snuck in from the study-abroad experience. Luckily, he'd been an embracing support since they met freshman year and managed to bring her back to her usual cheerful (albeit serious and academic) self. Within a day or two, they were able to enjoy the rest of the trip.

Meredith was busy planning her semester, with a roster of literature courses, interspersed with an intense extracurricular schedule: editing for one of the school papers, tutoring freshman English, and peer mentoring at the school's LGBTQ resource center. After her experience abroad, she was newly inspired to support other trans students. She was also starting to think about life after college, considering a career in journalism.

She caught me up on what life was like after her vaginoplasty. The summer before college ended up being tough because of her recovery period and missing all her friends' summer parties before going off to college. The dilation schedule (needed to prevent the newly formed vagina from closing) was time-consuming and difficult—four times a day at the beginning. The surgical recovery also temporarily took away her biggest coping skills—running and biking—at a time when she needed them the most. Despite all of this, she's glad she had the surgery in the summer instead of during freshman year at college, which would have been nearly impossible to manage without taking a semester off and falling behind.

After arriving on campus for the first time, Meredith found herself in an existential crisis. She had focused so much of her life and time on studying and getting into college, and now she was there—at a top school with endless opportunities. She didn't know what to do next and wondered what that meant. She started to experience depression, and student health services connected her with a new on-campus therapist. Within a few months, she began to feel better. She attributes this mostly to settling into classes and finding her new goal—to become a journalist and excel in storytelling. I brought up that the average person might wonder if any of the depression was related to gender or her surgery, but she explained that those didn't really cross her mind at the time. Her transness at that point seemed like nothing compared to the existential crisis of what to do with her life and career. It's an important reminder that trans people are people, and that not everything comes back to the fact that they're transgender. She was dealing with typical high-achiever stress and a family genetic history that put her at a higher risk of depression. Therapy helped, and as she felt better, her grades soared, and in February of her freshman year, she met her boyfriend, Jason.

She had been asked out countless times in middle and high school, including by boys who reminded her that they didn't care she was trans. She went on dates with a few guys in high school, but never felt at ease before Jason. Though she didn't like talking to people about it at the time, she said she's more open postsurgery to talking about how the hang-up was not feeling content with her body, and her genitals specifically. The vaginoplasty allowed her to feel fully at home in her own skin. This freedom to feel like herself and also be intimate with Jason was an intensely affirming experience for her. She let me know she was aware of the comments in the media that trans women who have a vaginoplasty after early pubertal suppression had lack of sensation and could not orgasm. She wanted readers to know that this was not the case for her. "Honestly, I think our sex life is healthier and more enjoyable than many of my cisgender friends, who struggle with sex for all kinds of reasons." Her comment was well taken—I've had cisgender patients who struggle with sexuality for all kinds of reasons: body insecurities, depression, anxiety, not knowing how to navigate romantic and sexual relationships, not having had appropriate sex education, and a range of traumatic experiences ranging from emotional to physical.

As we spoke more about her life at college and her friend group, she told me she wanted to emphasize something important she had been thinking about recently. Up until college, she didn't have any trans friends. She was lucky to have a stalwart and loving network of affirming friends and family, but they were all cisgender. Toward the end of freshman year of college, she formed a group of tight-knit friends who are all trans women.

"I'm not the kind of person who thinks you need to have the same experience as someone to know what they're going through, but there is an experience of talking about things that cis people may see as uncertainty that is easier to talk to trans people about." For example, she found it easier to talk to her trans friends about insecurities in how she presented and whether she was "feminine enough." While cisgender people may see that as uncertainty around who she is or whether she is "really" trans, her trans friends got it and could talk to her without weird conversations about whether she thought she was actually cisgender (she did not). Another thing they had spoken about recently was how friendships with boys could be difficult. Her group of trans girlfriends all happen to be straight, and they have worried that if they make friends with boys, it may be perceived as flirting, then the relationship could be tainted by transphobia. Having talked through this with her trans girlfriends, Meredith now feels much more comfortable with those anxieties and has developed a strong group of male friends she's not sure she would have been able to get close with had she not had her trans girlfriends for support.

Having this friend network had given her a feeling of ease and relief, something she hoped she could give others through her new volunteering at the LGBTQ resource center on campus. Giving back in this way helped her deepen her sense of pride and community, which made her feel more grounded, confident, and self-assured.

Toward the end of our conversation, Meredith told me that she would need to run because her computer science class was starting soon. I let her know how heartwarming it was to see her grow up into such a strong young adult, and a big smile came across her face. She let me know she was excited for the book and for people to understand that being trans was complicated in today's society, but also beautiful, and that trans people can and do have amazing lives.

Nicole's and Meredith's relationships got me thinking more about something parents often ask me about their trans kids' futures—how are dating and family building likely to evolve as more people are open and accepting of gender diversity? To talk about this a bit more, I reached out to my friend Chris Mosier. Chris is an absolute phenom triathlete. He is a seven-time member of Team USA and a three-time national champion. He's also a strong advocate for transgender people like himself. Because of his advocacy, he sadly is a victim of a steady stream of antitrans hate messages. I wanted to know more about what his support system was like and how he handled it all. Chris let me know that at the end of the day his partner is his number one support. The two met in college, prior to Chris's transitioning. The partner had come to visit Chris's roommate, who turned to Chris and said, "You two aren't going to like each other; please be nice." The roommate was wrong, and the two started dating. His partner ended up being looped in closely with the queer community around them, which really helped Chris feel more comfortable and accepted, so that over time he could open up more about who he was. After two years, they moved in together. A few years later, they got a rabbit who lived with them, for thirteen years. The house sounded adorable, with ultimately three bunnies who had free range to hop around the house (Chris taught me that bunnies can use litter boxes). Chris and his partner have now been together for twenty-one years and are considering fostering children sometime in the near future.

In talking about romantic relationships, Chris made an important point for parents to know. We talked about how many parents worry about their children finding love and families if they are openly trans—afraid they won't find partners. And that's just not true—there are people everywhere who love and support trans people. But to be in a strong romantic relationship, one truly needs to love oneself. And to be able to do that is no small feat when you're surrounded by voices saying that trans people aren't worthy of love and basic human rights. Chris got an important message from his mom when he came out to her. Though she was scared, there was one big takeaway: she loved him, supported him, and just wanted him to be happy. As he explained, "She loves and supports me. Even when not fully understood, I've felt loved and supported." This kind of support helps young people have the self-esteem they need to be able to navigate through life and connect well with others, and it's an extraordinary power parents can give their children. Though Chris does a lot of work fighting for his community, he also has a lot to love about himself in addition to loving his transness: his athletic success, his strong long-term relationship—and of course his nerdy love of magic tricks and "amazing mustache." The power to love oneself is one of the greatest gifts a parent can give a child, and it's a gift that allows people to have thriving relationships with others.

SAM

Because Sam was doing well and didn't really have any concerns around gender, they stopped seeing me regularly. However, it turned out they developed some symptoms of OCD, so they started seeing a therapist who focused on the evidence-based treatment for this: exposure and response-prevention therapy. About a year after our most recent meeting, I saw that Sam had popped up on my clinic schedule. I walked out to see them and their mom in the waiting room. It was clear Sam had gone through a growth spurt and was now much taller than their mom. They were wearing gym shorts with paint stains on them (they later told me the paint was from working on a set for a school play) and a *Little Mermaid* T-shirt (the new live-action version had just come out). They had grown their braids long and held them back from their face with a ponytail. When we got back to my office, Sam and their mom both grabbed the putty tins I keep in my office for people to fidget with, before sitting down next to each other on the couch.

I told them it was great to see them and asked what brought them back. It turned out it had nothing to do with gender. Sam was still settled in the same nonbinary gender identity as before. They had been admitted to a high school for the arts, where they were focusing on set design and hoping to work in theater in the future. They had a great set of friends who were also passionate about the arts and were loving school. But the OCD hadn't gotten better. Therapy helped, but their obsessive concerns about handwashing and things being contaminated hadn't gone away. When I looked down at their hands, I could see that they were chapped from the way constant handwashing can clear away the natural oils that keep skin from damaging.

Their therapist had told them it was time to consider psychiatric medication to help with the OCD in addition to therapy. Having heard that some psychiatrists in their area pathologized trans identities and wouldn't just focus on Sam's OCD, they called and made an appointment with me instead. We talked about the risks, benefits, and side effects of fluoxetine (also called Prozac) and started the medication that same day. Sam, who had friends who had gone through gender-affirming medical care, smiled a bit after I sent the prescription. "It's funny that you could just talk about the side effects with us and prescribe it instead of going through a whole series of therapy sessions the way my friends did for estrogen." It was a stinging comment, but I knew it came from a place of wanting to push my thinking. It wasn't the first time the point had crossed my mind. All medications have risks and side effects. Some of them are severe (even the commonly prescribed antibiotic penicillin, for instance, can cause a rare side effect called Stevens-Johnson syndrome, in which a person's skin can detach). But the letter requirement prior to prescribing a medication was unique for gender-affirming medical care.

His comment got me reflecting again on where the field of pediatric gender medicine may evolve over the next decade or so. In the realm of adult gender medicine, standards had clearly moved away from the so-called gatekeeping model, and prescribers no longer required extensive mental health assessments prior to starting gender-affirming hormones. Estrogen and testosterone were prescribed in much the same way other medications—such as fluoxetine—were prescribed. People were told about the risks, benefits, and potential side effects. They asked any questions they had, then they received a prescription. In general, this seemed to be going well for many thousands of patients around the world. In pediatric gender medicine, however, the politics had forced things even further in the opposite direction. With the threat of legislation and political violence, most pediatric gender clinics had become even more strict in the assessments they conducted prior to considering pubertal suppression or gender-affirming hormones. In all honestly, it was impossible for me to predict how things would evolve over the next few years, but I turned to Sam and let him know that I understood where he was coming from. I could understand how people could feel invalidated and stigmatized when their receiving medications was held to a different standard from when cisgender people received medications.

Sam nodded at me, signaling that they felt I had heard them. They let me know that they were happy to see me again. They loved their new therapist, who was helping with their OCD, but the recent antitrans talk in the media was starting to really stab at their mental health. Though they didn't see a clear connection between that and the OCD, they noticed their OCD was getting worse. I shared that stress in general can do that.

"I'm confident in who I am, and I'm so lucky that my mom has always accepted me. I hate it, but the news is messing with how I think about myself. I know that there's nothing wrong with me, but seeing on the news every day that there is some-thing new . . . it's driving me crazy."

I told Sam we could make our medication check-in appoint-ments more frequent and longer, so that we could keep tabs on how the news was impacting him and ways it might be tricking his mind into impacting his self-esteem. I felt myself holding back tears as we wrapped up our conversation, the sides of my mouth tensing as I tried to hold back a frown. Even these kids who were doing so well, who were protected by loving families and affirmed, were being impacted, simply by the words of people who didn't even live in the same state. It was heartbreaking, and it wasn't fair.

KYLE

As with Sam, I had also been meeting with Kyle periodically to manage the antidepressant medication he took. I met with him several months after his top surgery, when he was finally healed. He wanted to tell me about a family dinner he had recently had with his mom and dad. They had gone out to their favorite Italian restaurant near their house. The dinner was pretty mundane—they talked about school, what was new with friends, and what movie they were going to watch together that night (the *Hocus Pocus* sequel won out). What was so remarkable to Kyle was that the dinner felt *so normal*. He couldn't believe how different life was now from how it was years ago. When he was still hiding his trans identity from his family, he felt that their relationship was strained. They didn't really know him. He was in so much pain that he felt he needed to keep to himself.

Now, he felt so much more connected to them. They had made huge progress in working to understand his experience, religiously attending the parent support groups that had connected them with other parents of trans youth. Their work made him feel loved, accepted, understood, and validated. His parents, of course, had always loved him deeply, but this process opened up the pathway for them to all come together, truly see one another, and be able to express that love in a way it could be received. Kyle had been so consumed by his gender dysphoria before that he hadn't even thought about what it would be like to have an open, connected relationship with his parents, and he described the feeling as a comforting warmth deep in his soul that kept him feeling grounded and connected. He could talk to them about gender-related things when they came up, but mostly he was able to just be a normal boy and talk to them the way other kids talk to their parents.

For most appointments, I leave parents a few minutes at the end to chat with me one-on-one, while their child waits in the waiting room. Rosa and Juan let me know that everything was going well from their perspective too. Despite their worries going into Kyle's top surgery, they described being relieved to see how much more confident and comfortable Kyle was with himself after. He had given me permission to tell them about how he felt at the recent dinner. When I told them, they said they felt the same way—that they finally were able to be a family that just talked like other families. The huge chasm they used to feel between themselves and Kyle was rapidly closing. It hurt them that he had suffered so much before, and they were grateful for the support groups and health care providers who had helped them with their own journey of coming to understand and support Kyle. "It was hard for us. We've always just wanted what was best for him, but we didn't know what it was. It took us time, and we're happy that everyone supported us and helped us come along this journey, too." Rosa reached toward the tissues I keep on the side table next to the couch. She sniffled, straightened her posture, and shook my hand before she and Juan walked back out to the waiting room to get Kyle. I watched Kyle bump into his mom affectionately as they headed toward the elevators to go back home.

FREE TO BE

Wanting to talk more about how transitioning can deepen relationships, I reached out to another close friend and trans role model, Dallas Ducar. Dallas is a licensed nurse practitioner whom I met when I was doing my residency at Harvard Medical School, and we've stayed in close touch over the years. She is the founding CEO of Transhealth—a pioneering organization advancing trans health and providing care to over two thousand patients. She holds faculty appointments at Columbia University, the University of Virginia, and Massachusetts General Hospital. She's been a strong voice in the realm of trans health care, with op-eds published in *Newsweek* and the *Boston Globe*, and she served on the transition team for the attorney general of Massachusetts. In recent years, she's frequently been called upon for her expertise, as lawmakers try to understand what kinds of policies are most likely to improve public health.

I caught up with her when she was in-between meetings in Washington, DC, and noticed she had taken on the DC look—a professional long black dress, gold earrings that matched her gold necklace, and a GLAAD pin fixed to her clothes. She spoke with the passion and clarity of someone who has navigated the political system. After she caught me up on some recent polling numbers and her thoughts on where antitrans policies are headed (she's optimistic), the conversation turned more personal. I told her I wanted to talk about queer love and relationships in the book, and like Chris, she explained that coming out and having the ability to be her authentic self, and to bring her whole self to a relationship, made a huge difference. It allowed her to better connect with people and feel truly known. All types of relationships became easier after she transitioned: dating, friendships, and those with family. Though she loves her life and doesn't regret her path, she did lament the years she lost in high school when she was hiding herself and missed out on being able to form deeper relationships because she didn't feel safe being her true open self. She went on, "Isn't that what every parent wants—for their kid to be known, and understood, and have meaningful long love with people who truly understand them?"

Dallas and I closed our conversation talking about how the upcoming election was going to reveal a lot about our country and the politicization of identity. As I finish writing this book, politicians in the United States are starting to indicate their intentions to run in the presidential primaries. I see regular headlines about what *politicians think* about transgender youth and their families. I suspect that when this book comes out, trans kids will be a major topic in our political debates. My plea to everyone is to make sure this debate about trans youth doesn't *exclude the voices of trans youth*. It's far too easy for conversations about trans kids, their rights, and their medical care to become intellectualized and separated from the actual lives and experiences of these young people. Before making up your mind about these kids, or policies that impact them, go meet them—hear what they have to say. Hear about their lives and experiences. I hope the stories some of them have so generously shared for this book will add the human experience to some of these conversations.

As we've seen, gender is complex, and it brings up emotions in all of us. It's important to listen to those emotions and unpack what they mean. Perhaps in reading this, you've come to a more nuanced understanding of your own gender identity—with its complex web of relationships to gender roles, feelings about your body, and transcendent feelings of gender that are hard to put into words. You may have come to understand what difficult gender-related experiences in your own past—from harassment, to discrimination, to being forced into gender boxes—have a tendency to bring up emotions for you. The work to unpack the complexities of our own genders, how society's handling of gender has impacted us, and how gender and society intersect is tough work, but it's essential—now more than ever. Fighting the temptation to oversimplify, as many politicians have done, and instead jumping into the complexity, will allow us all to not just support trans youth, but also better understand ourselves, as we continue through a world that is inevitably impacted by gender.

My sincerest hope is that by expanding your knowledge of the science, medicine, and politics of gender, you'll feel empowered to more fully dive in and understand what's at stake in today's gender wars. I hope you feel empowered to advocate for a society where sound, well-researched gender science is trusted, and where people of all gender identities and experiences are acknowledged, respected, and treated with kindness and dignity. My dream is that we'll all be equipped with the information and inspiration to stand up for transgender children and move our communities toward a healthier, more nuanced, and loving gendered world. And most important, I hope you'll become a powerful advocate for making sure that children—your own or those in your life—are free to be who they truly are, in all their beautiful unique gender diversity.

Acknowledgments

First and foremost, I want to thank the incredible trans people (youth and adults both) who so kindly spoke with me for this book and shared their experiences. We are so privileged to be able to hear their stories. I am also eternally grateful to my patients, who constantly push me to think more critically about gender and our gendered society. I want to thank the many incredible trans scholars who have generously educated me over the years. To name just a few: Maddie Deutsch, Alex Chen, Susan Stryker, Chase Strangio, Julia Serano, Florence Ashley, Jules Gill-Peterson, Brynn Tannehill, Alejandra Caraballo, Kinnon MacKinnon, Erin Reed, Marci Bowers, Colt St. Amand, Nick Gorton, Nate Sharon, Ari Drennen, Gillian Branstetter, Dallas Ducar, and Tony Ferraiolo. I'm indebted to Dana Simpson for the beautiful illustration for chapter 2. My mentees have also had a huge impact on me, and I'm eternally grateful to Brett Dolotina in particular for their tireless research and writing to advance trans youth mental health. I'm also in debt to my writing mentors Drs. Lisa Sanders, Suzanne Koven, Chase Anderson, and Wednesday Martin for constantly pushing me to be a better writer and storyteller. And to some of the incredible physicians who selflessly provided feedback on the technical portions of this book: Drs. Michelle Forcier, Norman Spack, and Blair Peters. I'm also thankful to my other physician and psychology mentors, Drs. Alex Keuroghlian, Andrés Martin, Diane Ehrensaft, Christy Olezeski, Gerrit van Schalkwyk, Zheala Qayyum, Susan Kashaf, Christopher Ruser, Nancy Angoff, Chris Brady, Caitlin Costello, and Anne Glowinski. And of course a huge thank-you to Todd Shuster, Jack Haug, Lauren Liebow, and Daniella Cohen at Aevitas Creative for helping me to conceptualize this book, and to my tireless editor, Stephanie Hitchcock at Atria, for her brilliance and patience. My friends and family were also incredible supports, especially Beth Shields, Tiffany Bradshaw, Ziad Reslan, and Glenn Felder, who graciously provided feedback. Last but not least, thank you to my Samoyed, Kodi, for booping me when I needed to step away from the keyboard to take him on walks.

Resources

MENTAL HEALTH CRISIS SERVICES

The Trevor Project: Provides mental health crisis support for LGBTQ youth. Crisis supports are available over the phone (866-488-7386), through SMS (678678), or online chat (https://www.thetrevorproject.org/webchat).

988: The U.S. national mental health crisis line is available throughout the country, and you can specifically request a counselor who focuses on supporting LGBTQ people.

Trans Lifeline: A peer support phone service (877-565-8860) run by trans people for trans and questioning peers. "Call us if you need someone trans to talk to, even if you're not in crisis or if you're not sure you're trans."

READING ABOUT GENDER-AFFIRMING MEDICAL CARE

UCSF Gender-Affirming Health Program: This program (http://transcare.ucsf.edu/guidelines) has in-depth information on gender-affirming medical interventions for medical providers and also has useful "overviews" of various treatments geared toward what patients need to know.

World Professional Association for Transgender Health Standards of Care 8 (WPATH SOC): At the time of writing, these are the most recent clinical care guidelines from WPATH, written for health care and mental health providers (https://www.wpath.org/soc8).

Endocrine Society Guidelines: These are similarly written for health care and mental health providers (https://www.endocrine.org/clini cal-practice-guidelines/gender-dysphoria-gender-incongruence).

SERVICES FOR FAMILIES AND COMMUNITIES

Gender Spectrum: A national organization committed to the health and well-being of gender diverse children and teens through education and support for families, and training and guidance for educators, medical and mental health providers, and other professionals (https://genderspectrum.org/). They offer countless resources including templates for gender support plans at school and online support groups for parents of transgender and gender diverse youth.

PFLAG: A national organization of LGBTQ+ people and their loved ones, with many parents of LGBTQ youth. There are local chapters throughout the country, which can provide community and support (https://pflag.org/about-us/).

LEGAL AND ADVOCACY ORGANIZATIONS

Transgender Legal Defense and Education Fund: A legal organization focused on supporting transgender and gender diverse people, including through their Name Change Project, which provides pro bono legal name change services for low-income people in need.

The Transgender Law Center: Maintains a legal help desk to help people understand the rights of transgender people under the law (https://transgenderlawcenter.org/resources/).

Lambda Legal: A national LGBTQ legal advocacy organization that maintains a help desk that can provide general information and resources related to discrimination based on gender identity and expression (https://lambdalegal.org/helpdesk/).

ADDITIONAL READING

Becoming Nicole: The Extraordinary Transformation of an Ordinary Family **by Amy Ellis Nutt**
This book takes an in-depth dive into the life of Nicole Maines, who is interviewed throughout, and her family's experience.

Being Jazz: My Life as a (Transgender) Teen **by Jazz Jennings**
Jazz Jennings came to national prominence at age five, when she and her family opened up their life on the TLC show *I Am Jazz*. This memoir brings readers into Jazz's life as a transgender teen, while encouraging them to accept themselves, live an authentic life, and embrace their own truths.

Found in Transition: A Mother's Evolution during Her Child's Gender Change **by Paria Hassouri**
In this memoir, pediatrician Paria Hassouri vulnerably discussed the experience of her daughter coming out as trans and many of the common challenges parents face through this experience.

He/She/They: How We Talk About Gender and Why It Matters **by Schuyler Bailar**
This comprehensive book by Harvard NCAA Division I swimmer Schuyler Bailar uses storytelling and the art of conversation to give readers the essential language and context to better

understand gender, as we reckon with unprecedented attacks on transgender Americans.

Histories of the Transgender Child by Jules Gill-Peterson
Though a more academic read, this landmark book challenges the myth that the phenomenon of children coming out as trans is "new"—documenting the experiences of transgender children, and their access to gender-affirming medical care, throughout the twentieth century.

Trans Bodies, Trans Selves: A Resource by and for Transgender Communities edited by Laura Erickson-Schroth
A comprehensive, reader-friendly, 728-page guide for transgender people, with each chapter written by transgender and gender-expansive authors.

Transgender History: The Roots of Today's Revolution by Susan Stryker
Written by one of the foremost trans academics of today, *Transgender History* takes a chronological approach to transgender history from the mid-twentieth century to today.

Whipping Girl: A Transsexual Woman on Sexism and the Scapegoating of Femininity by Julia Serano
A landmark book by biologist and trans activist Julia Serano detailing her personal experiences to reveal the ways in which fear, suspicion, and dismissiveness toward femininity shape our attitudes toward trans women, as well as gender and sexuality as a whole.

Glossary

Agender: A gender identity term describing when people do not identify with gender as part of their identity.

Asexual: A term that describes a person who experiences little or no sexual attraction toward others.

Binding: Wearing tight clothing or using other mechanisms to minimize the appearance of chest tissue.

Bisexual: A sexual orientation that describes a person who is emotionally and/or sexually attracted to both men and women.

Bottom surgery: A colloquial term describing gender-affirming genital surgeries (e.g., vaginoplasty or phalloplasty).

Cisgender: An umbrella term describing when one's gender identity aligns in a traditional sense with one's sex assigned at birth.

Differences of sexual development: An umbrella term for the many ways in which various domains of sex (e.g., chromosomes, external genitalia, internal genitalia) do not neatly align. Some also use the synonymous term *intersex*.

Gender-affirming hormones: Hormonal treatments (generally estrogen or testosterone) used to help one's physical body align with one's gender identity.

Gender dysphoria: A concept defined in the American Psychiatric Association's *Diagnostic and Statistical Manual of Mental Disorders* as a clinically significant distress resulting from an incongruence between one's gender identity and one's sex assigned at birth.

Gender expression: The way one presents to the world in a gendered way (e.g., a dress may be thought of as a feminine gender expression and a suit may be thought of as a masculine gender expression).

Gender identity: One's psychological sense of one's own gender (e.g., male, female, nonbinary, or another gender).

Gender incongruence: A term used by the World Health Organization's International Classification of Diseases to describe when one's gender identity does not align with one's sex assigned at birth.

Gender minority: An adjective used to describe a person who is not cisgender.

Gonadotropin-releasing hormone analogs: Medications that temporarily pause a person's puberty. These medications are sometimes called blockers, puberty blockers, or pubertal suppression.

Intersex: An umbrella term for the many ways in which various domains of sex (e.g., chromosomes, external genitalia, internal sex organs) do not neatly align. Some also use the synonymous term *differences of sexual development*.

Metoidioplasty: A surgical procedure that involves releasing ligaments attached to the clitoris to create a phallus.

Minority stress: A model that explains the ways in which societal stigma can lead to mental health challenges for minoritized populations.

Nonbinary: A term used when one does not identify as strictly male or strictly female. They may identify with both gender identities, neither, or somewhere in between.

Orchiectomy: A surgical procedure that involves removal of the testes.

Pansexual: A romantic/sexual orientation term that describes a person who is emotionally and/or physically attracted to people of all gender identities.

Phalloplasty: A surgical procedure that involves creation of a penis.

Puberty blocker: A medication that temporarily pauses a person's puberty. These medications are technically called gonadotropin-release hormone analogs, or sometimes GnRHa for short.

Queer: An umbrella term often used to describe the sexual and gender minority community at large, encompassing lesbian, gay, bisexual, transgender, questioning, intersex, and asexual communities.

Sex assigned at birth: The sex that is listed on someone's birth certificate, usually male or female, and generally based on the appearance of external genitalia observed at birth. In the past, some have used *natal sex* or *birth sex* as synonyms.

Sexual minority: An adjective used to describe someone who is not heterosexual.

Sexual/romantic orientation: Describes the types of people toward whom one has physical, emotional, and/or romantic attachments.

Thyroid chondroplasty: A surgery that involves minimizing the appearance of an Adam's apple.

Top surgery: A colloquial term for gender-affirming surgery of the chest.

Transgender: An umbrella term describing when one's gender identity does not align, based on societal expectations, with one's sex assigned at birth.

Transsexual: An older term that is often considered pejorative to describe when one's gender identity does not align with one's sex assigned at birth. Some use this term to specifically refer to transgender people with a desire for gender-affirming medical or surgical interventions and do not consider the term pejorative.

Vaginoplasty: A surgical procedure that involves the creation of a vagina.

Vulvoplasty: A surgical procedure that involves creation of a vulva.

Notes

1. In the Crossfire: Meet Meredith, Kyle & Sam

11 **But that same research also:** T. D. Steensma et al., "Factors Associated with Desistence and Persistence of Childhood Gender Dysphoria: A Quantitative Follow-Up Study." *Journal of the American Academy of Child & Adolescent Psychiatry* 52 (6) (2013): 582–90.

14 **In fact, in one of the studies:** K. R. Olson, "Prepubescent Transgender Children: What We Do and Do Not Know," *Journal of the American Academy of Child & Adolescent Psychiatry* 55 (3) (2016): 155–56.

20 **Though negative experiences with parents:** S. Luthar and R. Prince, "Developmental Psychopathology," in *Lewis's Child & Adolescent Psychiatry: A Comprehensive Textbook*, 5th ed., ed. A. Martin, M. H. Bloch, and F. R. Volkmar (Philadelphia: Wolters Kluwer, 2018).

22 **Not until years later:** J. L. Turban et al., "Association between Recalled Exposure to Gender Identity Conversion Efforts and Psychological Distress and Suicide Attempts among Transgender Adults," *JAMA Psychiatry* 77 (1) (2020): 68–76.

23 **One Canadian study of:** R. J. Watson, J. F. Veale, and E. M. Saewyc, "Disordered Eating Behaviors among Transgender Youth: Probability Profiles from Risk and Protective Factors," *International Journal of Eating Disorders* 50 (5) (2017): 515–22.

24 **After leaving the hospital:** James Lock and Daniel Le Grange, *Treatment Manual for Anorexia Nervosa: A Family-Based Approach*, 2nd ed. (New York, NY: Guilford Press, 2013).

24 **Only recently have eating disorder therapists:** S. M. Hartman-Munick et al., "Eating Disorder Screening and Treatment Experiences in Transgender and Gender Diverse Young Adults," *Eating Behaviors* 41 (2021): 101517.

31 **In a sample of eighty-five children:** J. R. Rae et al., "Predicting Early-Childhood Gender Transitions," *Psychological Science* 30 (5) (2019): 669–81.

2. A Child by Any Other Name: Understanding the Language of Gender

36 **This kind of body diversity:** M. Blackless et al., "How Sexually Dimorphic Are We? Review and Synthesis," *American Journal of Human Biology: The Official Journal of the Human Biology Association* 12 (2) (2000): 151–66.

37 **Later in the 1940s:** Cydney Grannan, "Has Pink Always Been a 'Girly' Color?," *Encyclopaedia Britannica*, https://www.britannica.com/story/has-pink-always-been-a-girly-color.

42 **Therapy with the goal of:** American Academy of Child & Adolescent Psychiatry, "Policy Statement on Conversion Therapy," accessed September 28, 2023, https://www.aacap.org/AACAP/Policy_Statements/2018/Conversion_Therapy.aspx.

45 **In a recently published study:** T. E. Charlesworth and M. R. Banaji, "Patterns of Implicit and Explicit Stereotypes III: Long-Term Change in Gender Stereotypes," *Social Psychological and Personality Science* 13 (1) (2022): 14–26.

48 **Research shows that attempts to:** J. L. Turban et al., "Association between Recalled Exposure to Gender Identity Conversion Efforts and Psychological Distress and Suicide Attempts among Transgender Adults," *JAMA Psychiatry* 77 (1) (2020): 68–76.

49 **For kids like Kyle:** E. W. Diemer et al., "Gender Identity, Sexual Orientation, and Eating-Related Pathology in a National Sample of College Students," *Journal of Adolescent Health* 57 (2) (2015): 144–49.

50 **In describing the typical audience reaction:** Julia Serano, *Whipping Girl: A Transsexual Woman on Sexism and the Scapegoating of Femininity*, 2nd ed. (Emeryville, CA: Seal Press, 2007).

51 **A 2022 study from the Pew Research Center:** "About 5 Percent of Young Adults in the U.S. Say Their Gender Is Different from Their Sex Assigned at Birth," Pew Research Center, 2022, https://www.pewresearch.org/fact -tank/2022/06/07/about-5-of-young-adults-in-the-u-s-say-their-gender -is-different-from-their-sex-assigned-at-birth/.

59 **In 2018, researchers from the University of Texas at Austin:** S. T. Russell et al., "Chosen Name Use Is Linked to Reduced Depressive Symptoms, Suicidal Ideation, and Suicidal Behavior among Transgender Youth," *Journal of Adolescent Health* 63 (4) (2018): 503–5.

61 **It's technically a mental health diagnosis:** American Psychiatric Association, *Diagnostic and Statistical Manual of Mental Disorders*, 5th ed., *Text Revision (DSM-5-TR)*, (Arlington, VA: American Psychiatric Publishing, 2022).

61 **In reality, being transgender is merely a healthy:** Ibid.

63 **In fact, research shows that transgender people:** S. James et al., *The Report of the 2015 US Transgender Survey* (Washington, DC: National Center for Transgender Equality, 2016).

63 **When we recently looked at data:** J. L. Turban et al., "Sex Assigned at Birth Ratio among Transgender and Gender Diverse Adolescents in the United States," *Pediatrics* 150 (3) (2022): e2022056567.

3. Gender Foundation:
The Biology of Diverse Gender Identities

68 **I'd also be remiss not to highlight:** K. R. Olson et al., "Gender Identity 5 Years After Social Transition," *Pediatrics* 150 (2) (2022).

72 **Wanting to stop this from happening to other people:** J. Colapinto, *As Nature Made Him: The Boy Who Was Raised as a Girl* (New York, Harper-Collins, 2001).

73 **In 2005, Columbia University psychologist:** H. F. Meyer-Bahlburg, "Gender Identity Outcome in Female-Raised 46,XY Persons with Penile

Agenesis, Cloacal Exstrophy of the Bladder, or Penile Ablation," *Archives of Sexual Behavior* 34 (4) (2005): 423–38.

75 **Twin studies related to gender identity have suggested:** M. Diamond, "Transsexuality among Twins: Identity Concordance, Transition, Rearing, and Orientation," *International Journal of Transgenderism* 14 (1) (2013): 24–38.

75 **In 2012, a team of researchers published a study:** G. Heylens et al., "Gender Identity Disorder in Twins: A Review of the Case Report Literature," *Journal of Sexual Medicine* 9 (3) (2012): 751–57.

76 **Some researchers have theorized that these epigenetic changes:** K. Ramirez et al., "Epigenetics Is Implicated in the Basis of Gender Incongruence: An Epigenome-Wide Association Analysis," *Frontiers in Neuroscience* 15 (2021): 1074.

77 **In a 2005 review article:** T. Mazur, "Gender Dysphoria and Gender Change in Androgen Insensitivity or Micropenis," *Archives of Sexual Behavior* 34 (4) (2005): 411–21.

77 **Odiele, for example, told the *Guardian*:** Aaron Hicklin, "Intersex and Proud: Model Hanne Gaby Odiele on Finally Celebrating Her Body," *Guardian*, April 23, 2017, https://www.theguardian.com/fashion/2017/apr/23/intersex-and-proud-hanne-gaby-odiele-the-model-finally-celebrating-her-body.

78 **A 2005 review article found that among such people:** P. T. Cohen-Kettenis, "Gender Change in 46,XY Persons with 5α-Reductase-2 Deficiency and 17β-Hydroxysteroid Dehydrogenase-3 Deficiency," *Archives of Sexual Behavior* 34 (4) (2005): 399–410.

80 **This gave the patient more time to reflect:** L. M. McGee et al., "Pubertal Suppression and Surgical Management of a Patient with 5-Alpha Reductase Deficiency," *Urology*, S0090-4295.

81 **In their 1959 paper in the journal *Endocrinology*:** C. H. Phoenix et al., "Organizing Action of Prenatally Administered Testosterone Propionate on the Tissues Mediating Mating Behavior in the Female Guinea Pig," *Endocrinology* 65 (3) (1959): 369–82.

82 **In his book *Different*, primatologist Frans de Waal:** Frans de Waal, *Different: Gender through the Lens of a Primatologist* (New York: Norton, 2022).

83 **The results were apparent from the first two:** J. Thornton, J. L. Zehr, and M. D. Loose, "Effects of Prenatal Androgens on Rhesus Monkeys: A Model System to Explore the Organizational Hypothesis in Primates," *Hormones and Behavior* 55 (5) (2009): 633–44.

84 **However, these early studies did establish:** M. Diamond and H. K. Sigmundson, "Sex Reassignment at Birth: Long-Term Review and Clinical Implications," *Archives of Pediatrics & Adolescent Medicine* 151 (3) (1997): 298–304.

84 **In 2019, an international team of researchers:** J. G. Theisen et al., "The Use of Whole Exome Sequencing in a Cohort of Transgender Individuals to Identify Rare Genetic Variants," *Scientific Reports* 9 (1) (2019): 1–11.

86 **They found that results for trans people:** H. Berglund et al., "Male-to-Female Transsexuals Show Sex-Atypical Hypothalamus Activation When Smelling Odorous Steroids," *Cerebral Cortex* 18 (8) (2008): 1900–1908.

86 **A 2021 review of all the different neuroimaging studies:** A. Frigerio, L. Ballerini, and M. Valdes Hernandez, "Structural, Functional, and Metabolic Brain Differences as a Function of Gender Identity or Sexual Orientation: A Systematic Review of the Human Neuroimaging Literature," *Archives of Sexual Behavior* 50 (8) (2021): 1–24.

87 **Similar genetic studies:** K. Servick, "Study of Gay Brothers May Confirm X Chromosome Link to Homosexuality," *Science*, November 17, 2014, https://www.science.org/content/article/study-gay-brothers-may-confirm-x -chromosome-link-homosexuality-rev2.

4. It's Always the Mom: The Pseudoscience of Blaming Parents and Social Environments

99 **She was so sold:** Lawrence J. Friedman, *The Lives of Erich Fromm: Love's Prophet* (New York: Columbia University Press, 2013).

99 **In 1948, she famously proposed:** F. Fromm-Reichmann, "Notes on the Development of Treatment of Schizophrenics by Psychoanalytic Psychotherapy," *Psychiatry* 11 (3) (1948): 263–73.

99 **The idea that mothers were responsible:** S. S. Kety et al., "Mental Illness in the Biological and Adoptive Families of Adopted Schizophrenics," *American Journal of Psychiatry* 128 (3) (1971): 302–6.

104 **In 1964, he published the book:** Bernard Rimland, Ph.D., *Infantile Autism: The Syndrome and Its Implications for a Neural Theory of Behavior* (Philadelphia: Jessica Kingsley Publishers, 1964).

104 **Most notably, in a 1977 study:** S. Folstein and M. Rutter, "Infantile Autism: A Genetic Study of 21 Twin Pairs," *Journal of Child Psychology and Psychiatry* 18 (4) (1977): 297–321.

105 **In his 1975 book:** Robert Stoller, *Sex and Gender: The Development of Masculinity and Femininity* (New York: Routledge, 1968).

105 **In their 1995 book:** Kenneth Zucker and Susan Bradley, *Gender Identity Disorder and Psychosexual Problems in Children and Adolescents* (New York: Guilford, 1995).

106 **In 1991, two researchers from St. Luke's Roosevelt Hospital Center:** S. Marantz and S. Coates, "Mothers of Boys with Gender Identity Disorder: A Comparison of Matched Controls," *Journal of the American Academy of Child & Adolescent Psychiatry* 30 (2) (1991): 310–15.

107 **Of the four who had a history of hospitalization:** Zucker and Bradley, *Gender Identity Disorder.*

107 **In a 1988 paper, a psychiatrist named Leslie Lothstein:** L. Lothstein, "Self-Object Failure and Gender Identity," in *Frontiers in Self Psychology*, ed. A. Goldberg (Hillsdale, NJ: Analytic, 1988).

108 **They found that the moms of the transgender girls:** Zucker and Bradley, *Gender Identity Disorder.*

108 **In her 2016 book on the topic:** Alison Gopnik, *The Gardener and the Carpenter: What the New Science of Child Development Tells Us about the Relationship between Parents and Children* (New York: Farrar, Straus and Giroux, 2016).

110 **In 1993, Zucker and Bradley set out to test this hypothesis:** K. J. Zucker et al., "Physical Attractiveness of Boys with Gender Identity Disorder," *Archives of Sexual Behavior* 22 (1) (1993): 23–36.

110 **A few years later, the same researchers conducted an identical study:** S. R. Fridell et al., "Physical Attractiveness of Girls with Gender Identity Disorder," *Archives of Sexual Behavior* 25 (1) (1996): 17–31.

112 **The therapists thought moms being too close:** H. F. Meyer-Bahlburg, "Gender Identity Disorder in Young Boys: A Parent- and Peer-Based Treatment Protocol," *Clinical Child Psychology and Psychiatry* 7 (3) (2002): 360–76.

112 **They thought that spending too much time:** Ibid.

112 **Those efforts didn't work:** J. L. Turban et al., "Association between Recalled Exposure to Gender Identity Conversion Efforts and Psychological Distress and Suicide Attempts among Transgender Adults," *JAMA Psychiatry* 77 (1) (2020): 68–76.

113 **Dr. Lisa Littman, an obstetrician-gynecologist:** L. Littman, "Parent Reports of Adolescents and Young Adults Perceived to Show Signs of a Rapid Onset of Gender Dysphoria," *PLoS One* 13 (8) (2018): e0202330.

114 **In an interview with the *Economist*:** "Why Are So Many Teenage Girls Appearing in Gender Clinics?," *Economist*, September 1, 2018, https://www.economist.com/united-states/2018/09/01/why-are-so-many-teenage-girls-appearing-in-gender-clinics.

118 **Analyzing a sample of over sixteen thousand transgender adults:** J. L. Turban et al., "Age of Realization and Disclosure of Gender Identity among Transgender Adults," *Journal of Adolescent Health* 72 (6) (2023): 852–59.

119 ***Wall Street Journal* columnist Abigail Shrier published:** Abigail Shrier, "Opinion: When Your Daughter Defies Biology," *Wall Street Journal*, January 26, 2019, https://www.wsj.com/articles/when-your-daughter-defies-biology-11546804848.

119 **Shrier went on to write *Irreversible Damage*:** Abigail Shrier, *Irreversible Damage: The Transgender Craze Seducing Our Daughters* (Washington, DC: Regnery, 2020).

119 **The *Economist* ran similar pieces:** "Why Are So Many Teenage Girls Appearing in Gender Clinics?," *Economist*.

119 **Every major medical organization:** J. L. Turban, K. L. Kraschel, and I. G. Cohen, "Legislation to Criminalize Gender-Affirming Medical Care for Transgender Youth," *JAMA* 325 (22) (2021): 2251–52.

119 **The American Psychological Association issued a statement:** American Psychological Association et al., "CAAPS Position Statement on Rapid Onset Gender Dysphoria (ROGD)," 2021, https://www.caaps.co/rogd-state ment.

120 **The journal editors required Dr. Littman to revise the paper:** L. Littman, "Correction: Parent Reports of Adolescents and Young Adults Perceived to Show Signs of a Rapid Onset of Gender Dysphoria," *PLoS One* 14 (3) (2019): e0214157.

120 **Soon after the 2018 paper was published:** Brooke Sopelsa, "Brown Criticized for Removing Article on Transgender Study," NBC News, September 5, 2018, https://www.nbcnews.com/feature/nbc-out/brown-university-criticized -over-removal-transgender-study-n906741. Accessed: September 30, 2023.

120 **Ben Shapiro wrote a piece for the *Daily Wire*:** Ben Shapiro, "A Brown University Researcher Released a Study about Teens Imitating Their Peers by Turning Trans. The Left Went Insane. So Brown Caved," *Daily Wire*, August 28, 2018, https://www.dailywire.com/news/brown-university-researcher-re leased-study-about-ben-shapiro.

122 **As one transgender teen in a focus group once told me:** J. Turban et al., "Ten Things Transgender and Gender Nonconforming Youth Want Their Doctors to Know," *Journal of the American Academy of Child & Adolescent Psychiatry* 56 (4) (2017): 275–77.

5. Puberty Blockers: Buying Time

127 **In one seminal study by Dr. Ryan's research team:** C. Ryan et al., "Family Acceptance in Adolescence and the Health of LGBT Young Adults," *Journal of Child and Adolescent Psychiatric Nursing* 23 (4) (2010): 205–13.

128 **On the other hand, she found that expressing love:** Family Acceptance Project, "Supportive Families, Healthy Children: Helping Families with Lesbian, Gay, Bisexual, & Transgender Children," San Francisco State

University, accessed October 2, 2023, https://familyproject.sfsu.edu/sites/ default/files/documents/FAP_English%20Booklet_pst.pdf.

128 **A team of researchers reported:** C. Yu et al., "Marching to a Different Drummer: A Cross-Cultural Comparison of Young Adolescents Who Challenge Gender Norms," *Journal of Adolescent Health* 61 (4) (2017): S48–S54.

132 **In a 2016 study of eighteen hundred trans people:** S. Peitzmeier et al., "Health Impact of Chest Binding among Transgender Adults: A Community-Engaged, Cross-Sectional Study," *Culture, Health & Sexuality* 19 (1) (2017): 64–75.

133 **For example, the American Society of Plastic Surgeons highlighted:** American Society of Plastic Surgeons, Procedural Statistics Release, February 19, 2024, https://www.plasticsurgery.org/documents/News/Statistics /2022/plastic-surgery-statistics-report-2022.pdf.

134 **Dr. Spack came into the conference room:** P. Cohen-Kettenis and S. H. van Goozen, "Pubertal Delay as an Aid in Diagnosis and Treatment of a Transsexual Adolescent," *European Child & Adolescent Psychiatry* 7 (4) (1998): 246–48.

136 **A series of papers in the 1980s showed:** F. Comite et al., "Short-Term Treatment of Idiopathic Precocious Puberty with a Long-Acting Analogue of Luteinizing Hormone-Releasing Hormone: A Preliminary Report," *New England Journal of Medicine* 305 (26) (1981): 1546–50.

140 **Because clinical guidelines, set forth by the Endocrine Society:** W. C. Hembree et al., "Endocrine Treatment of Gender-Dysphoric/Gender-Incongruent Persons: An Endocrine Society Clinical Practice Guideline," *Journal of Clinical Endocrinology & Metabolism* 102 (11) (2017): 3869–903.

140 **and the World Professional Association for Transgender Health:** E. Coleman et al., "Standards of Care for the Health of Transgender and Gender Diverse People, Version 8," *International Journal of Transgender Health* 23 (suppl. 1) (2022): S1–S259.

144 **Most have linked this intervention to better mental health:** Two studies had neutral findings. A study from the United Kingdom by Carmichael et al. followed forty-four adolescents with gender dysphoria before and after

puberty blockers and found no change in their mental health. They note that this lack of a statistically significant finding could reflect their small number of participants or that they had no control group. Psychological distress and self-harm tend to increase over the course of adolescence, and that the mental health of those on puberty blockers in their study didn't worsen could indicate that the treatment helped. A second study from Texas by Kuper et al. found improvements in mental health when they combined the effects of puberty blockers and gender-affirming hormones, but when they looked at puberty blockers alone, they found no change. This could again reflect that the sample size of those who received puberty blockers only was much smaller. A third study by Hisle-Gorman et al. looked at health care utilization following gender-affirming medical care and found increased mental health care utilization and use of psychiatric medications after care, though they note that this may have represented responsible ongoing care due to closer contact with the health care system during treatment with gender-affirming care, rather than a worsening of mental health.

144 **These studies include some from the original Dutch clinic:** A. L. de Vries et al., "Puberty Suppression in Adolescents with Gender Identity Disorder: A Prospective Follow-Up Study," *Journal of Sexual Medicine* 8 (8) (2011): 2276–83; and A. I. van der Miesen et al., "Psychological Functioning in Transgender Adolescents before and after Gender-Affirmative Care Compared with Cisgender General Population Peers," *Journal of Adolescent Health* 66 (6) (2020): 699–704.

144 **a study from the United Kingdom that found:** R. Costa et al., "Psychological Support, Puberty Suppression, and Psychosocial Functioning in Adolescents with Gender Dysphoria," *Journal of Sexual Medicine* 12 (11) (2015): 2206–14.

144 **and a study from our group when I was at Harvard Medical School:** J. L. Turban et al., "Pubertal Suppression for Transgender Youth and Risk of Suicidal Ideation," *Pediatrics* 145 (2) (2020).

145 **One of the best studies to look at this question:** Costa et al., "Psychological Support, Puberty Suppression, and Psychosocial Functioning in Adolescents with Gender Dysphoria," 2206–14.

148 **There had been one study of the impact of puberty blockers:** A. S. Staphorsius et al., "Puberty Suppression and Executive Functioning: An

fMRI-Study in Adolescents with Gender Dysphoria," *Psychoneuroendocrinology* 56 (2015): 190–99.

150 **In a 2017 study in the *Journal of Adolescent Health*:** L. Nahata et al., "Low Fertility Preservation Utilization among Transgender Youth," *Journal of Adolescent Health* 61 (1) (2017): 40–44.

151 **Another study published in 2020 in the journal *JAMA Pediatrics*:** K. C. Pang et al., "Rates of Fertility Preservation Use among Transgender Adolescents," *JAMA Pediatrics* 174 (9) (2020): 890–91.

151 **Suzanne worried about this because some studies:** K. Wierckx et al., "Sperm Freezing in Transsexual Women," *Archives of Sexual Behavior* 41 (5) (2012):1069–107; and K. Wierckx et al., "Reproductive Wish in Transsexual Men," *Human Reproduction* 27 (2) (2012): 483–87.

151 **Other studies of transgender youth also showed:** D. Chen et al., "Attitudes toward Fertility and Reproductive Health among Transgender and Gender-Nonconforming Adolescents," *Journal of Adolescent Health* 63 (1) (2018): 62–68.

152 **it is marketed by the company to work for a year:** E. Pine-Twaddell, R. S. Newfield, and M. Marinkovic, "Extended Use of Histrelin Implant in Pediatric Patients," *Transgender Health* 8 (3) (2023): 264–72, https://doi.org/10.1089/trgh.2021.0130.

6. Choosing Puberty: Estrogen & Testosterone

158 **It's so small, in fact, that it sneaks through the membranes:** C. M. Revankar et al., "A Transmembrane Intracellular Estrogen Receptor Mediates Rapid Cell Signaling," *Science* 307 (5715) (2005): 1625–30.

161 **In one study from the Netherlands:** C. J. M. de Blok et al., "Breast Development in Transwomen after 1 Year of Cross-Sex Hormone Therapy: Results of a Prospective Multicenter Study," *Journal of Clinical Endocrinology & Metabolism* 103 (2) (2018): 532–38.

161 **An additional study of 69 trans women:** C. J. de Blok et al., "Sustained Breast Development and Breast Anthropometric Changes in 3 Years of Gender-Affirming Hormone Treatment," *Journal of Clinical Endocrinology & Metabolism* 106 (2) (2021): e782–e790.

161 This is in contrast with studies of cis women: V. Swami et al., "The Breast Size Rating Scale: Development and Psychometric Evaluation," *Body Image* 14 (2015): 29–38.

162 For trans women who do go through testosterone puberty: Z. Paige L'Erario, "Voice Training Is a Medical Necessity for Many Transgender People," *Scientific American*, September 19, 2022, https://www.scientificamerican.com/article/voice-training-is-a-medical-necessity-for-many-transgender-people/.

163 In 2020, researchers from Amsterdam published: S. Bungener et al., "Sexual Experiences of Young Transgender Persons during and after Gender-Affirmative Treatment," *Pediatrics* 146 (6) (2020).

169 In the same way that there are many different gender identities: K. C. Pang et al., "Long-Term Puberty Suppression for a Nonbinary Teenager," *Pediatrics* 145 (2) (2020).

171 The hospital had a policy of rooming people based on their gender identity: W. Acosta et al., "Identify, Engage, Understand: Supporting Transgender Youth in an Inpatient Psychiatric Hospital," *Psychiatric Quarterly* 90 (2019): 601–12.

173 They were particularly wary of some: J. L. Turban, K. L. Kraschel, and I. G. Cohen, "Legislation to Criminalize Gender-Affirming Medical Care for Transgender Youth," *JAMA* 325 (22) (2021): 2251–52.

7. Gender Surgery

185 In a qualitative study published: J. E. Mehringer et al., "Experience of Chest Dysphoria and Masculinizing Chest Surgery in Transmasculine Youth," *Pediatrics* 147 (3) (2021).

8. The Science of Gender Politics: Bathrooms, Sports & Legislating Medicine

197 At this time of writing, the American Civil Liberties Union: "Mapping Attacks on LGBTQ Rights in U.S. State Legislatures," American Civil

Liberties Union, accessed October 7, 2023, https://www.aclu.org/legisla tive-attacks-on-lgbtq-rights.

201 **In 2019, researchers from the Harvard School of Public Health:** G. R. Murchison et al., "School Restroom and Locker Room Restrictions and Sexual Assault Risk among Transgender Youth," *Pediatrics* 143 (6) (2019).

202 **They found that trans-inclusive facility policies:** A. Hasenbush, A. R. Flores, and J. L. Herman, "Gender Identity Nondiscrimination Laws in Public Accommodations: A Review of Evidence regarding Safety and Privacy in Public Restrooms, Locker Rooms, and Changing Rooms," *Sexuality Research and Social Policy* 16 (1) (2019): 70–83.

203 **Advocates for women's sports:** E. J. Staurowsky et al., *Chasing Equity: The Triumphs, Challenges, and Opportunities in Sports for Girls and Women* (New York: Women's Sports Foundation, 2020).

204 **The same strategy is being recycled today:** Jack Turban, "Opinion: What the Anti-Trans Movement Is All About," CNN, April 24, 2023, https:// www.cnn.com/2023/04/24/opinions/anti-trans-rhetoric-strategy-turban/ index.html.

205 **One columnist summed up the social conservative opinion:** Abigail Shrier, "Opinion: Joe Biden's First Day Began the End of Girls' Sports," *Wall Street Journal,* January 22, 2021, https://www.wsj.com/articles/joe-bidens -first-day-began-the-end-of-girls-sports-11611341066?mod=article_inline.

207 **It harkened back to a past:** Andrew Lawrence, "How the 'Natural Talent' Myth Is Used as a Weapon against Black Athletes," *Guardian*, October 2, 2018.

208 **In December 2023:** Larry Neumeister, "Court Revives Lawsuit over Connecticut Rule Allowing Trans Girls to Compete in School Sports," *Washington Post*, December 15,2023, https://www.washing tonpost.com/sports/2023/12/15/connecticut-transgender-student-athletes /7c425f22-9b7f-11ee-82d9-be1b5ea041ab_story.html.

209 **The vast majority couldn't name a single one:** David Crary and Lindsay Whitehurst, "Lawmakers Can't Cite Local Examples of Trans Girls in Sports," Associated Press, March 3, 2021.

209 **In a public statement explaining his veto:** Lindsay Whitehurst and Sam Metz, "Utah Governor Vetoes Transgender Sports Ban, Faces Override," Associated Press, March 22, 2022.

209 **State lawmakers largely ignored his remarks:** Adam Edelman, "Utah Legislature Overrides Governor Veto of Transgender Sports Ban Bill," NBC News, March 25, 2022, https://www.nbcnews.com/politics /politics-news/utah-legislature-overrides-governors-veto-transgender -sports-ban-bill-rcna21459.

209 **Families of trans youth in Utah:** Natalie Prieb, "Utah Families Sue Utah over Transgender Sports Ban," *Hill*, June 3, 2022.

211 **In a 2023 commentary in the peer-reviewed journal:** B. Hamilton, F. Guppy, and Y. Pitsiladis, "Comment on: 'Transgender Women in the Female Category of Sport: Perspectives on Testosterone Suppression and Performance Advantage,'" *Sports Medicine*, September 20, 2023, 1–6.

211 **A 2017 survey of over seventeen thousand youth:** "Play to Win: Improving the Lives of LGBTQ Youth in Sports: A Special Look into the State of LGBTQ Inclusion in Youth Sports," Human Rights Campaign, 2017, https://assets2.hrc.org/files/assets/resources/PlayToWinFINAL.pdf?_ga= 2.79969047.1693573134.1530650153- 950807199.1530034427.

212 **It turns out that trans youth have lower:** Behdad Navabi et al., "Pubertal Suppression, Bone Mass, and Body Composition in Youth with Gender Dysphoria," *Pediatrics* 148 (4) (2021).

212 **In an editorial in the journal *Pediatrics*:** L. K. Bachrach and C. M. Gordon, "Bone Health among Transgender Youth: What Is a Clinician to Do?," *Pediatrics* 148 (4) (2021).

213 **In 2022, a team of researchers published a study:** M. D. Hoffmann et al., "Associations between Organized Sport Participation and Mental Health Difficulties: Data from over 11,000 US Children and Adolescents," *PLoS One* 17 (6) (2022): e0268583.

213 **When Kentucky introduced a bill to ban trans youth:** Erin Kelly, "What's Next for Kentucky Student Who Testified against Trans Sports Bill," Spectrum News 1, June 13, 2022, https://spectrumnews1.com/ky/bowling-green

/news/2022/06/13/what-s-next-for-a-kentucky-student-who-testified -against-trans-sports-bill.

213 **Fischer was the only known transgender athlete:** Moriah Balingit, "Kentucky's Lone Transgender Athlete Can't Play on the Team She Helped Start," *Washington Post*, August 25, 2022, https://www.washingtonpost.com/ education/2022/08/25/fischer-wells-trans-athlete-kentucky/.

214 **The theory was first popularized by:** I. H. Meyer, "Minority Stress and Mental Health in Gay Men," *Journal of Health & Social Behavior* 36 (1) (1995).

214 **Later in 2012, psychologists noted:** Michael L. Hendricks and Rylan J. Testa, "A Conceptual Framework for Clinical Work with Transgender and Gender Nonconforming Clients: An Adaptation of the Minority Stress Model," *Professional Psychology: Research and Practice* 43 (5) (2012): 460.

218 **They hoped that if Carolyn:** Alice Evans, "Trans Conversion Therapy Survivor: 'I Wanted to Be Cured So Asked to Be Electrocuted,'" BBC News, August 23, 2019, https://www.bbc.com/news/uk-49344152.

218 **Gender identity conversion therapy is different:** Florence Ashley, "Transgender Conversion Practices: A Legal and Policy Analysis," in *Banning Transgender Conversion Practices* (Vancouver: University of British Columbia Press, 2022).

219 **In 2019, our research group published a study:** J. L. Turban et al., "Psychological Attempts to Change a Person's Gender Identity from Transgender to Cisgender: Estimated Prevalence across US States 2015," *American Journal of Public Health* 109 (10) (2019): 1452–54.

219 **As mentioned in the parent-blaming chapter:** H. F. Meyer-Bahlburg, "Gender Identity Disorder in Young Boys: A Parent- and Peer-Based Treatment Protocol," *Clinical Child Psychology and Psychiatry* 7 (3) (2002): 360–76.

220 **In the book *Irreversible Damage*:** Abigail Shrier, *Irreversible Damage: The Transgender Craze Seducing Our Daughters* (Washington, DC: Regnery, 2020).

221 **In 2019, our research group published a study:** J. L. Turban et al., "Association between Recalled Exposure to Gender Identity Conversion Efforts and Psychological Distress and Suicide Attempts among Transgender Adults," *JAMA Psychiatry* 77 (1) (2020): 68–76.

222 **Sadly, some people appear to be practicing conversion:** "Policy Statement on Conversion Therapy," American Academy of Child & Adolescent Psychiatry, 2018, https://www.aacap.org/aacap/Policy_Statements/2018/Conversion_Therapy.aspx.

223 **Given that federal circuit courts now have divergent:** John Fritze, "Religion vs. LGBTQ+ Rights: Supreme Court Weighs 'Conversion Therapy' Bans for Minors," *USA Today*, October 9, 2023, https://www.usatoday.com/story/news/politics/2023/10/09/supreme-court-conversion-therapy-ban-lgbtq-minors-tingley/71037697007/.

224 **In February of 2020, the South Dakota House:** Shoshana Dubnow, "South Dakota Lawmakers Pass Bill Blocking Transgender Minors from Receiving Surgery," ABC News, February 1, 2020, https://abcnews.go.com/Politics/south-dakota-lawmakers-pass-bill-blocking-transgender-minors/story?id=68648384.

224 **I wrote a piece about the proposed law:** Jack Turban, "What South Dakota Doesn't Get about Transgender Children," *New York Times*, February 6, 2020, https://www.nytimes.com/2020/02/06/opinion/transgender-children-medical-bills.html.

224 **when the bill failed to pass the South Dakota Senate:** Tim Fitzsimons, "South Dakota's Trans Health Bill Is Effectively Dead, Opponents Say," NBC News, February 10, 2020, https://www.nbcnews.com/feature/nbc-out/south-dakota-s-trans-health-bill-effectively-dead-opponents-say-n1134356.

224 **As of September 2023, the Human Rights Campaign:** "Map: Attacks on Gender Affirming Care by State," Human Rights Campaign, accessed November 3, 2023, https://www.hrc.org/resources/attacks-on-gender-affirming-care-by-state-map.

224 **In his opinion, Trump-appointed Alabama judge:** Tierney Sneed, "Judge Blocks Alabama Restrictions on Certain Gender-Affirming Treatments for Transgender Youth," CNN, May 14, 2022, https://www.cnn.com/2022/05/14/politics/judge-blocks-alabama-transgender-law/index.html.

225 **Gender-affirming medical care also isn't experimental:** Jack Turban, "The Evidence for Trans Youth Gender-Affirming Medical Care," *Psychology Today*, January 24, 2022, https://www.psychologytoday.com/us/blog/

political-minds/202201/the-evidence-trans-youth-gender-affirming-med
ical-care.

225 **Among them is a recent study of 315 adolescents:** D. Chen et al., "Psychosocial Functioning in Transgender Youth after 2 Years of Hormones,"
New England Journal of Medicine 388 (3) (2023): 240–50.

226 **Most aren't aware that every relevant major medical organization:**
J. L. Turban, K. L. Kraschel, and I. G. Cohen, "Legislation to Criminalize
Gender-Affirming Medical Care for Transgender Youth," *JAMA* 325 (22)
(2021): 2251–52.

226 **In the United Kingdom:** "Puberty Blockers: Under 16s 'Unlikely to Be
Able to Give Informed Consent,'" BBC, December 1, 2020, https://www
.bbc.com/news/uk-england-cambridgeshire-55144148.

226 **A later case in the United Kingdom emphasized this point:** Hugo
Greenhalgh, "UK Court Rules in Favour of Parental Consent in Trans
Treatment Row," Reuters, March 26, 2021, https://www.reuters.com/article/
britain-lgbt-legal/uk-court-rules-in-favour-of-parental-consent-in-trans
-treatment-row-idUSL8N2LO43Q.

226 **a higher court there also ultimately overturned:** Haroon Siddique,
"Appeal Court Overturns UK Puberty Blockers Ruling for Under-16s,"
Guardian, September 17, 2021, https://www.theguardian.com/society/2021/
sep/17/appeal-court-overturns-uk-puberty-blockers-ruling-for-under-16s
-tavistock-keira-bell.

226 **In one qualitative study of 273 parents:** K. M. Kidd et al., "'This
Could Mean Death for My Child': Parent Perspectives on Laws Banning
Gender-Affirming Care for Transgender Adolescents," *Journal of Adolescent
Health* 68 (6) (2021): 1082–88.

227 **Soon after politicians in Texas:** Jack Turban, "Opinion: Texas Officials
Are Spreading Blatant Falsehoods about Medical Care for Transgender
Kids," *Washington Post*, March 21, 2022, https://www.washingtonpost.com/
opinions/2022/03/01/texas-ken-paxton-greg-abbott-misinformation-trans
gender-medical-care/.

9. An Eye on the Future: How Gender and Society Will Continue to Evolve

233 **A *Pride* story about them quoted Nate:** Taylor Henderson, "*Supergirl Star Nicole Maines Is Dating TikTok Cosplayer Nate Weir*," *Pride*, January 3, 2022, https://www.pride.com/celebrities/2022/1/03/supergirl-star-nicole-maines-dating-tiktok-cosplayer-nate-weir.

234 **Her comment reminded me of a 2022 concurring opinion:** Quint Forgey and Josh Gerstein, "Justice Thomas: SCOTUS 'Should Reconsider' Contraception, Same-Sex Marriage Rulings," *Politico*, June 24, 2022, https://www.politico.com/news/2022/06/24/thomas-constitutional-rights-00042256.

243 **Some of them are severe:** E. Y. Lee, C. Knox, and E. J. Phillips, "Worldwide Prevalence of Antibiotic-Associated Stevens-Johnson Syndrome and Toxic Epidermal Necrolysis: A Systematic Review and Meta-Analysis," *JAMA Dermatology* 159 (4) (2023): 384–92, https://doi.org/10.1001/jamadermatol.2022.6378.

Index

Page numbers in *italics* refer to illustrations. Page numbers beginning with 253 refer to resources and glossary.

social media as important lifeline
for, 118*n*
see also homosexuals,
homosexuality; nonbinary
identities; transgender
identities; transgender youth
Linehan, Marsha, 49*n*
Lipitor (atorvastatin), 149
Little Mermaid (play), 242
Little Shop of Horrors (musical), 156
Littman, Lisa, 113–15, 117, 119, 120
lordosis, 81, 82
Lothstein, Leslie, 107–8
luteinizing hormone (LH), 135, 136*n*

Maines, Nicole, 199–200, 201, 202,
232–35, 240
Maines, Wayne, 199
Mark (Katie's father), 92, 94, 95, 104
marriage equality, 88, 121, 217, 234
Mary (autistic girl), 102, 103
Massachusetts, 202, 247
mastectomies, gender-affirming, 183,
185, 186
see also top surgeries
masturbation, 163
Matrix, The (film), 217
Mayo Clinic, 71
Melissa (nonbinary youth), 46–48,
49, 61–62
Mercer, Carolyn, 218, 219
Meredith (transgender girl), 9–21,
26, 31, 67–69, 80, 107, 108, 151–53,
155–58, 163–65, 195–96, 235–40
fear of puberty in, 16–17, 18, 156
gender therapy sought by, 14–15,
18, 147, 172, 191–92, 194
hormone therapy of, 158, 159–62,
165–68, 169, 176, 191
puberty blockers and, 17–19, 147, 148,
149, 150, 152–53, 155, 157, 165, 167*n*

social transition of, 14, 15–16, 17
sports participation of, 212
vaginoplasty of, 191–95, 196,
236–37, 238
metoidioplasty, 258
Meyer, Ilan, 214
Meyer-Bahlburg, Heino, 73–74,
219–20, 221
Millett, Kate, 70
minority stress model, 214–17
definition of, 259
Money, John, 69–70, 71–73, 75*n*, 76,
81, 84*n*
Moran, Maddie, 78–80
Morphosis, Maddy (Daniel Truitt),
64–65, *64*
Mosier, Chris, 232, 240, 247
Mosser, Scott, 186*n*
mothers, blaming of, *see* parents,
blaming of
mounting, 81, 82, 83

Nate (Nicole Maines's partner), 233
Nazis, 99, 103
negative expectations, 215–16
"neopronouns," 60
Netherlands, 17, 137, 161
neuroimaging studies, 85–86
New Delhi, India, 128
New England Journal of Medicine, 225
Newsweek, 247
New York Times, 3, 9, 224
NIH (National Institutes of
Health), 143–44, 188, 253
nonbinary, definition of, 259
nonbinary identities, 49*n*, 50–51,
57–58, 61, 64, 126, 132, 151, 167*n*,
168–70, 242
chest binding by, 132–33
gender-affirming medical care for,
133, 168–69, 186

"Pubertal Delay as an Aid in
Diagnosis and Treatment of
a Transsexual Adolescent"
(*European Child & Adolescent
Psychiatry* article), 134–38
puberty, 23, 31, 77, 123, 157
brain's role in, 124–25, 135–36
early-onset, 136, 148
hormones in, 78, 80, 126, 135–36,
156, 159, 160n, 161, 162, 186
nonbinary identities and distress
over, 169n
Sam's indifference toward, 124–27,
168, 169, 170
as source of fear and distress in
trans kids, 16–17, 18, 24, 123, 125, 126,
129, 131, 132, 133, 135, 140, 142, 156
Tanner staging in, 18, 27
puberty blockers, 5, 6n, 17–19, 26, 27,
31, 80, 124, 129, 133–37, 147, 155, 157,
163, 168, 192, 210, 238
bone density and, 18, 147, 157, 158,
169n, 212
brain development and, 148
definition of, 259
fertility issues and, 149–52, 165
GnRH analogs as, 135–36, 152n
implantation procedure for, 152–53
"informed consent" model for, 143,
144, 148
lack of double-blind studies on,
144–45
menopause-like symptoms of,
147–48
mental health benefits of, 137–38,
144, 145–46, 155–56, 225–26, 228
physical benefits of, 132, 133–34,
167n, 183n–84n, 186n
psychological assessment
requirements for, 138–41, 142–44,
148, 244

U.K. bans on, 226
"pushover mother" theory, 108

queer, definition of, 259
Quinn (nonbinary athlete), 210, 217

"rapid-onset gender dysphoria,"
113, 114, 115, 117, 119–21
rectovaginal fistula, 193
"refrigerator mother" theory, 102,
103, 104, 109
Regenerus, Mark, 121
Reimer, Brian, 70, 71–72, 75n
Reimer, David (Bruce/Brenda),
70–73, 74, 75n, 76, 77, 84n
Reimer, Janet, 70, 71, 72, 81
Reimer, Ron, 70, 71, 72, 81
"resilience factors," in minority
stress framework, 216–17
rhabdomyolysis, 149
rhesus monkeys, 82, 83, 84
Rimland, Bernard, 103–4
Rimland, Mark, 103–4
Risk and Protective Factors
for Suicide among Sexual
Minority Youth study, 59
Roe v. Wade, 205n, 225n
Rolling Stone, 71, 72
Romer v. Evans, 204n
Rosa and Juan (Kyle's parents),
22–23, 24, 171, 173–80, 181, 188,
189–90, 245–46
support group attended by, 172,
173–76, 245, 246
Ross, Angelica, 55–56, 232
Rothblatt, Martine, 217, 232
Royal Pains (TV series), 232
RuPaul's Drag Race (TV series),
64–65, *64*
Rutter, Michael, 104
Ryan, Caitlin, 127–29

vaginal stenosis, 193
vaginoplasty, 183, 191–95, 196, 236–37, 238
   definition of, 260
   dilation regimen for, 192–93, 194, 237
   hair removal before, 193, 196
   risks of, 193, 194
   techniques for, 192
Veronica (transgender woman), 134,
   138
V for Vendetta (film), 217
vocal cord surgeries, 162
Vogue, 76
Volkmar, Fred, 104, 109
Vrije University Medical Center,
   Center of Expertise on Gender
   Dysphoria at, 6, 137
Vulnerable Child Protection Act
   (HB1057), 224
vulvoplasty, 193*n*, 260

Wachowski, Lana and Lilly,
   217, 232
Wall Street Journal, 58, 119, 205
Wells, Fischer, 213
"When Your Daughter Defies
   Biology" (*WSJ* op-ed), 119
Whipping Girl (Serano), 50, 256

Wicked (musical), 116
Witherspoon Institute, 121
Wolfson, Evan, 88, 89
Women's Sports Foundation, 203
World Health Organization,
   International Classification of
   Diseases of, 62
World Professional Association
   for Transgender Health
   (WPATH), 140, 184*n*
World Professional Association for
   Transgender Health Standards
   of Care 8 (WPATH-SOC), 254
World War II, 88, 99

X (formerly Twitter), 207, 231

Yale Child Study Center, 104, 109
Yale University, 2, 3
   Cushing Center at, 3–4
Yearwood, Andraya, 205–8
Yellowjackets (TV series), 232, 233
youthtranscriticalprofessionals.org, 113
YouTube, 118

Zucker, Kenneth, 6, 105–6, 107, 108,
   110–11

About the Author

Jack Turban, MD, is a Harvard-, Yale-, and Stanford-trained child and adolescent psychiatrist and director of the Gender Psychiatry Program at the University of California, San Francisco (UCSF). He is an internationally recognized researcher and clinician whose expertise and research on the mental health of transgender youth have been cited in legislative debates and major federal court cases regarding the civil rights of transgender people in the United States. He is also a frequent contributor to the *New York Times*, the *Washington Post*, *Scientific American*, and more. He has appeared on numerous programs, including *The Daily Show with Trevor Noah* and *PBS NewsHour*.